THE PARADOX OF POWER AND WEAKNESS

SUNY series, Alternatives in Psychology
Michael A. Wallach, editor

THE
PARADOX
OF
POWER
AND
WEAKNESS

*Levinas and an
Alternative Paradigm
for Psychology*

George Kunz

STATE UNIVERSITY OF NEW YORK PRESS

Published by
State University of New York Press, Albany

© 1998 State University of New York

Printed in the United States of America

For information, address State University of New York Press,
State University Plaza, Albany, N.Y., 12246

Production by Cathleen Collins
Marketing by Patrick Durocher

Library of Congress Cataloging in Publication Data

Kunz, George, 1934 –
    The paradox of power and weakness : Levinas and an alternative
paradigm for psychology / George Kunz.
        p.   cm. — (SUNY series, alternatives in psychology)
    Includes bibliographical references and index.
    ISBN 0–7914–3889–9 (hardcover : alk. paper). — ISBN 0–7914–3890–2
(pbk. : alk. paper)
    1. Psychology—Philosophy.   I. Title.   II. Series
BF38.K85   1998
171′.8—dc21
                                                                97–40917
                                                                CIP

10 9 8 7 6 5 4 3 2 1

In memory of my parents
Violet Simons Kunz (1903-1958)
Hilary Michael Kunz (1905-1971)

To my wife, Margo, children,
Matt, Hannah, Simon, Greta, and Max,
and granddaughters, Elizabeth and Madeline

Hineni = "Here I am."
(Isaiah 6:8)

"How can we determine the hour of dawn, when the night ends and the day begins?"

"When from a distance you can distinguish between a dog and a sheep?" suggested one of the students.

"No," was the answer of the rabbi.

"Is it when one can distinguish between a figtree and a grapevine?" asked a second student.

"No."

"Please tell us the answer then," said the students.

"It is then," said the wise teacher, "when you can look into the face of a human being and you have enough light to recognize in him your brother. Up until then it is night and darkness is still with us."

Hasidic tale

Contents

Acknowledgments

The deep rural and religious values my parents gave their seven children must be acknowledged as the foundation for this work.

I wish to express gratitude to Margo, my wife, for her constant support: this book took twelve years of her patience and helpful suggestions in response to my frustrations and exuberances. I thank the members of the psychology department here at Seattle University, especially Steen Halling, Lane Gerber, Jan Rowe, and Kevin Krycka, for their support, and my friends in the philosophy department, especially James Risser and Patrick Burke, who introduced me to Levinas's work in 1981. Getting some released time from teaching by receiving two university awards, the Gaffney Endowed Chair and the McGoldrick Fellowship, shortened what would have otherwise taken many more years. Old gratitude goes to Fr. John Evoy, SJ, who introduced me to psychology, this ambiguous science I have loved so much since his Psy 100 class in 1952, and to all my teachers, especially the Jesuits at St. Francis Xavier Seminary, Mount Saint Michael's, Gonzaga, Marquette, and Seattle Universities. Gratitude also goes to Andy Giorgi in the graduate program in phenomenological psychology at Duquesne University, who stimulated my thinking from 1967 to 1971, with his articulation of the radical break from mainstream psychology through the insights of the phenomenologists. I acknowledge the inspiration of Bill Grace, director of the Center for Ethical Leadership, upon whose board of advisors I have had the honor to sit for several years. Thanks goes to the thousands of students who have listened to the gradual development of the ideas in this book. They called my ideas into question often by expressions of confusion and boredom as well as enthusiasm. I wish to thank the critical readers who slogged through rough drafts and suggested changes: Fr. Pat Carroll, SJ, Dan Clingaman, David Hostetler, Karen Lutz, and Betsy Warriner. Finally, I am indebted to the editorial reviewers for supporting my efforts: Richard Cohen, David Harrington, James Hatley, and Ron Shaffer.

Prologue

Introducing herself as Bernice, a woman about thirty-five stood confidently in front of my class of thirty college students. She described, a bit haltingly, but clearly and focused, her life as a resident of a L'Arche community, a group home for developmentally disabled people and their assistants. She explained how the residents and assistants cleaned the house together. When they finished, they fixed a nice Saturday lunch to celebrate getting the work done. These lunches were like the bigger celebrations she loved so much: the parties, the special occasions that seemed to occur at least once a week, on birthdays, holidays, church feastdays, any excuse to have a party. After Bernice spoke for about ten minutes, Cindy, an assistant who lived with her, asked for questions. A few students asked Bernice questions: How long had she lived at L'Arche? How many residents lived with her? How many assistants? What was her second favorite thing besides the celebrations?

She gave short and direct answers. Then Cindy got up and offered more details and history on the L'Arche communities. She told us how Jean Vanier, the son of a Canadian diplomat, once a navel officer and then a professor, founded in 1963–64 the first community in France, where he set up housekeeping with two mentally disabled men. Now in each one of over a hundred L'Arche houses in twenty countries around the world, about six disabled residents and three assistants live together, share the work, and celebrate community.

The simplicity, humility, patience and generosity expressed by both the residents and assistants *touched* the hearts of these psychology students. Jean Vanier calls this *touch*, "the secret." (I quote extensively from his talk in St. James Cathedral, Seattle, May 30, 1992.)

> The *secret* is . . . that we need each other, the weak and the strong. Obviously the weak need the strong. What is less easily understood is that the strong need the weak. That is the secret.

[M]any will come to L'Arche to serve the poor. And that is good. But then they will stay in our communities, because they have discovered that they are poor, that we all have a wound, that we are all vulnerable, that there is a broken part in each of us, . . . that we all have masks and a system of protection, hiding our vulnerability, . . . that inside all of us, there is a place where anger hides, and fear, and depression, maybe broken sexuality, a capacity to live and lock ourselves up into a world of dreams. That is the *reality* of all of us. We have a handicap. It's all of us . . . some it's more visible; others it's less. But the reality is there. We come to serve the poor. We discover, after a while, that *we* are the poor.

But then . . . then, there is another discovery, that the good news is not announced to those who serve the poor, but that it is announced to those who are poor, to those who are weak, those who, in their weakness, serve the strong. *Incredible power of the powerless.* You see, people who have power, maybe we seek them in order to receive some share of power. We seek somebody in power.

But people like the beautiful child, Innocent, have another power. (Vanier had spoken earlier in his talk about Innocent, an adolescent resident of a L'Arche community in the Ivory Coast.) There was an incredible beauty. She couldn't speak. She couldn't use her hands. Of course, the thing with Innocent was that she didn't touch or awaken what I would call our "ego," our need to prove. She didn't ask for knowledge. She didn't ask for power. She didn't ask for money or generosity. She only asked one thing, "Do you love me?"

Innocent was demanding, because she could do nothing by herself. She needed to be clothed. She needed to be brought to the toilet. She needed to be fed. She needed . . . , she needed . . . , obviously, she needed somebody to be there, to play with her. That's demanding. It's true, it's very demanding. So the mystery is always that the poor, the weak, the powerless are crying out. But frequently we do not want to hear the cry of the poor, because of many reasons: fear, other things to do, multiplicity of reasons. So the poor always disturb. Always disturb. They break our patterns, our programs. We have already decided what we want to do, and the cry of the poor comes to disturb. That's why we don't want to listen to it.

But at the same time, the mystery is that they do disturb, and they *awaken*. They don't just touch our hearts; they *punch* our hearts. You know people in pain; we can never be neutral to people in pain. It is the power of the powerless; the power of the weak. Innocent doesn't excite in our hearts a desire for power or wealth. She doesn't create inside of us fear, . . . of being hurt, or of being crushed. Her eyes, her littleness, and her trust, these seem to awaken something very deep in the human heart. The innocence of Innocent tells us who we are.

People come to discover the secret, the secret which obviously many do not know, because in many places there is that need to crush the weak. But that secret also is known in many, many places: that those who are powerless have a gift to give, to transform our hearts. The secret . . . that if we get close to those who are broken, according to our call, according to the gift of our hearts, according to our situation, if we get close to people who are powerless, people in need, people crying out. If we enter into relationship with them, not just . . . , not just doing something for them, but looking them in the eyes, entering into a relationship where we enter into them. If we do that, certainly we will touch our own pain. We will touch our own fears. That is why we need community, because we can do nothing all alone. We need to belong. We only know ourselves and each other when we live with our weaknesses.

I used to think I taught the most important lessons in my introduction to psychology course. But I only set the scene while others teach my students the essential concepts of the human psyche. The L'Arche residents teach these essentials. The children and mothers in the protective hospitality house, the homeless and hungry in the shelters and kitchens, the children they tutor in the local grade schools, the elders at the retirement home, the marginalized unregistered voters my students try to get connected up to the political process, all these people, and the students caring for each other, teach "the secret" Jean Vanier speaks about. This *secret* is the paradox of the *power of weakness*.

Although easily found in concrete lives revealed in the faces of others, this paradox is a secret because, as Vanier says, people do not want to know it. What an odd secret! Most secrets are what we want to know but other people keep them hidden. This secret is available to all, but many individuals and institutions do not want it to be known.

In my course, I expect each student to spend sixteen hours at one of five selected community agencies. In the beginning, some students complain that the volunteer requirement in service-learning will take too much time out of their busy schedules of school, work, and fun. At the end of the ten-week quarter, they nearly all say service-learning became the best part of the course. Although this punches my ego, I am grateful to my "fellow co-teachers," the ones who serve my students by being served by them, who teach by revealing their weakness, who inspire in my students a deeper self-understanding and appreciation of others. Students who still complain at the end of the course about the service assignment missed the secret because they had earlier begged off to take an easy placement, or insisted they could not do any volunteering, and I had no right to require it. I accept their demands but then watch them miss the secret of this paradox. Some complain because they simply refuse to be touched.

Reading periodically through the students' journals of service experiences, I am struck by their growth in maturity. Although they are often frustrated by the lack of motivation in some grade-schoolers, or low self-esteem in many shelter residents and soup kitchen visitors, or inefficiency in the bureaucracy of some providing agencies, or the deceit of some rip-off recipients, the secret slowly sinks in. They learn not only about the people and agencies with whom they work, but especially about themselves as human psyches, about the social myths concerning what is important in life and what is unimportant, about the paradox of weakness, about the inexorable call to all of us to care about others, about the secret that all of us need care, all of us.

But the postmodern world teaches my students other lessons, ones that compete with Jean Vanier's secret about the *power of weakness*: these are the lessons of the *power of power*, and the *weakness of weakness*. These competing lessons are carried by the diffuse and persistent voice of *cynicism* saying, "Get real. The weak are losers. Go for power. Avoid the weak. Think of yourself." These lessons dismiss Jean Vanier's insight that says, "There is a reality: we have a handicap, and as we serve the vulnerable we discover the *power of their weakness* to heal us." To be touched and shaken by this paradox is to be humbled. Cynicism, refusing to be humbled, denies this paradox and condemns it as hypocrisy. Cynicism insists the very nature of power can admit within itself only power; and that weakness is a cancer to be cut out, nothing more. Not only does it claim these logically self-evident truths, cynicism also demonstrates empirical evidence to prove that power empowers and weakness only weakens. Weakness, to the "realist," cannot be paradoxically powerful.

Every few months some pollster reports a new all-time high in American cynicism. While voter participation numbers, consumer confidence data, and public opinion surveys express less trust in leadership, people use their self-justified anger to complain about *the system* and to justify their own manipulation of *the system* to get what they can whenever they can. The target of cynicism is often government decision-makers, elected and appointed, authorities higher up in any corporate chains of command, people in professions that have influential power such as lawyers, doctors, teachers, religious ministers. Even while watching our language in this time of political correctness, there is an increase in cynicism about people of other ethnic groups, gender, economic class, religions, age, and other groups.

Cynicism misses the *secret*!

Cynicism shows itself in three general forms. The most obvious form of cynicism is the contemptuous *criticism* of others, accusing those others not only of incompetence and fraud, but even more of the hypocrisy of hiding self-interested motives behind phony claims of honesty. The sarcasm of the cynic, exposing the flaws of others, not only serves to demonstrate the cynic's own highly perceptive powers of observation and intelligent insight, but also cleanly separates the cynic from any hypocritical corruption about which he or she is so scandalized. Cynics need hypocrites to justify their cynicism.

The second form of cynicism is the subtle and not so subtle *manipulation* of the system. Cynics take advantage of others by using the system for their own gain and justify their manipulation by appealing to the principle that competitive advantage-taking is the rule of the game: we have to do it to others before they do it to us. Pragmatically working the system is even more cynical than criticizing the system. As manipulators, cynics need to justify their own hypocrisy.

The last but perhaps most illusory form of cynicism is the self-indulgent *consumption* of capricious wants, justified as "well-deserved rewards." The claim, "I owe it to myself," is often a judgment of the ingratitude and greediness of others as well as a justification for the cynic's own selfishness.

These cognitive, behavioral, and affective forms of cynicism (arrogant criticism, cunning manipulation, and self-indulgent consumption) are implicitly supported by the so-called *truths* of modern psychology: self-care, self-esteem, self-confidence, self-reliance, self-assertiveness, self-justification, self-gratification, self-love, self-whatever. Psychology has nearly deified the self, paradoxically by reifying it as a natural force. The implicit natural law of *self-interest* acts as the core principle upon which much of the social sciences are founded, just as *energy as force* is a core principle in physics.

While psychology has moved self-interest to the heart of its philosophical assumptions about the nature of the human, self-righteous self-interest has become the heart of cynicism. Ideological self-righteousness has infected psychological, political, and economic structures, as well as their respective sciences, and has thus contributed to the social disease of postmodern cynicism. Paul C. Vitz warned twenty years ago in *Psychology as Religion: The Cult of Self-Worship* (1977), of the self-destructiveness of ego-centrism in psychology.

But there is another secret. Peter Sloterdijk, in his classic book, *Critique of Cynical Reason* (1983/1987), tells us that the cynical consciousness through which we pretend to show superior intelligence, successful control, and self-rewarding satisfaction, is in fact an unhappy consciousness. Although our sophistication often frees us to self-justified deception, we are sad. Although we sometimes treat conventional morality with irony as applicable only for the stupid, we admit no evil intent, only discontent. We reluctantly admit that our cynical suspicion is the only realistic way of seeing and doing things. While we mourn our loss of innocence, we carry on tasks with the clearest of all enlightened justifications: "Everybody else is doing it." The inhabitants of postmodernity are well-off and miserable. Sloterdijk defines postmodern cynicism, our sophisticated knowledge combined with diffuse depression about our behavior, as "enlightened false consciousness" (1983/1987, p. 5). We accept short-term optimism and reject hope. Our manic drive for success buffers us against any self-reflection that admits this violence against ourselves and others. We feel trapped between our longing for the good and the demand to fight for survival by the rules of a *cynical reality* that has incorporated those necessities we wish we did not have to carry out (pp. 3–8). The secret of the *weakness of power* accompanies the secret of the *power of weakness*.

I sense the anxiety in my students launching adult careers and lives that promise these deep conflicts. They anticipate their own collaboration in economic and social structures and activities that will demand unethical but practical behavior. They acknowledge that their own complicity in competitive processes that overtly or covertly violate others will make them dislike themselves; yet they are resigned to perform these assigned jobs. Really, what else can they do? They long for situations where they can be inspired by the *simplicity, humility*, and *patience* they see in the residents and assistants of the L'Arche communities, the diners and servers at the soup kitchens, the mothers and protectors at the guarded shelters, and others in marginalized settings and those trying to help them. But they have difficulty imagining themselves in that track. They feel caught in the track promising other kinds of consciousness, behavior, and so-called "good life," the social demand of self-interest.

I notice that too frequently modern psychology cannot be of help to these students, but only part of their problem. Psychology is distinguished among sciences in its inability to explain to people their puzzles and confusions. It has tried to explain away its ineptitude by claiming it is only a young science. But the puzzles and confusions of the human psyche, its paradoxes, its self-contradictions are anomalies due to the paradigm of modern psychology rather than the mere errors and naivete of an immature science. Psychology will never solve its inherent anomalies if it remains committed to the natural scientific approach and to the presupposition that human behavior which is based solely on the force of self-interested needs.

While the philosophical presupposition that *the self is the center of the self* has been the firm foundation of psychology, it has encouraged an egocentrism that sabotages itself. The promise that personal self-empowerment would bring levels of happiness and hope has too often betrayed the students of the science. Psychology should look at those secrets, recently pointed out by Vanier and Sloterdijk, but known by the wise of all eras: *humbly serving, the self finds itself; empowering itself, it is vulnerable to losing itself.* Just as the vulnerability of the child, Innocent, challenged the power of her assistants, and humbled them, so the weakness of the psyche ought to challenge the power of psychology, humble it, and open its eyes to the paradoxes of the power of weakness and the weakness of power.

My intention is to encourage psychology to turn for help to the extraordinarily challenging philosophy of Emmanuel Levinas in order to question the old paradigm and point in a different direction. The central theme of his philosophy is that *although egocentric, the self transcends this tendency and desires what is radically other than itself, what cannot be comprehended, controlled, or consumed: the awesome otherness of the Other.*[1] On the one hand, trying to totalize and thus violate Others in its obsession with itself, the self destroys itself. On the other hand, responding responsibly to and for Others, those infinitely mysterious beings beyond the reach of the categories and manipulations of the self, the self finds its true self and joy. Paradoxically the self cannot alone, out of its own power, choose to transcend its own self-obsessed and self-sabotaging power; it is only called out of its weakness toward self destruction by the inherent goodness and vulnerability of Others.

Logically, in physical and natural terms, power cannot be weak and weakness cannot be powerful. But nearly everyone recognizes the ambiguous use of those terms in social interaction. The bullies are weak, and victims are powerful in attracting our compassion. The tyrant's abuse is weaker than the innocent's vulnerability. Levinas finds the basis for this

---

1. Following the lead of Alphonso Lingus, translator of *Totality and Infinity*, who writes, "With the author's permission, we are translating *'autrui'* (the personal Other, the you) by 'Other' " (p. 24n), I will capitalize the O of *Other* when the word refers to the *other person*.

seeming self-contradiction in reflecting on *proto-ethics*, on the metaphysical basis for ethical behavior. The bully, powerful in dominating others, is
ethically weak; and the innocent, weak in natural force, is ethically powerful. Levinas's descriptions of *totality and infinity* and *need and desire* define
the paradoxes attended to in this book—that self-interested power can
turn out to be the weakness of the powerful, and that persons weakened
by psychological, sociological, political, and economic powers find their
weakness to be the basis of their ethical power to call others to serve them
precisely because they cannot make demands on others.

I make no claim to absolute originality for myself or Levinas. These
paradoxes, obviously familiar to many readers, have deep roots in religious and cultural traditions. We find the paradox of the power of weakness expressed deeply and widely in history, for example, by the ancient
Jewish proverb, "Others' physical needs are my spiritual needs," and by
the modern poet, Toni Morison, "The function of freedom is to free someone else." We find the paradox of the weakness of power in St. Paul's bla-
tantly self-contradictory statement, "I do what I would not and would not
what I do," and in James Baldwin's, "People pay for what they do, and
still more, for what they have become. And they pay for it simply: by the
lives they lead." The following lines of the Bengali poet, Tagore, com-
posed as a kind of epigram, exemplify the paradoxical:

I slept and dreamt, that life was all joy.
I awoke and saw, that life was but service.
I served and understood, that service was joy.

Although the paradoxes of power and weakness both haunt us from
tradition and disturb us as we daily encounter our neighbor, there has
been either an amnesia in modern times or an ideological force serving a
vested interest urging us to hide these insights from ourselves. Levinas's
philosophy rediscovers not only the possibility of *radical altruism*, where
"the Other is the center of the self," but also finds it as the glory of the
human psyche. Because of our modern personal and social poverty of ethical responsibility, Levinas's philosophy, which is more radical than any
ethics of personal generosity, may seem extravagant to our eyes and ears.

My point will be that psychology must revisit this wisdom that seems
so foolish to our modern cynicism in order to deepen and broaden its
understanding of the human psyche. Being at the end of modernism but
not yet established to have its own name, postmodernism has a choice
between either deeper cynicism or higher hope founded on the ethical
responsibility of radical altruism. Psychology can contribute either way.

PART I

Psychology's Anomaly and an Alternative Paradigm

CHAPTER ONE

Radical Altruism

An Anomaly to Modern Psychology

A REAL DISTINCTION BETWEEN ALTRUISM AND SELF-INTEREST

My friend John (not his real name), a social worker, operates out of a tiny office of a health clinic in downtown Seattle. Many of his clients are homeless, jobless, familyless, addicted, and often have some form of psychopathology. Some have criminal records, and most have broken-down, sad lives. Others live in low-rent housing, such as low-income elderly, disabled and working people who survive on meager incomes and whose need for services might be temporary. John helps people get their welfare checks, a little medical care, food, a bed, whatever they need and he can find. With other advocates, he pesters city hall for affordable housing, less police harassment, and more dignity for those who have been pushed to the edges of our high-rise, high-tech, high-energy society.

Although John's family is the center of his life (he shares with his wife the care of their young boys), he sacrifices lots of time, money, and energy he could otherwise spend on himself and his own for people whom he sees in his office, or whom he seeks out in shabby rooms and under viaducts and in packing crates behind warehouses. Each one represents for him an individual with dignity worthy of respect and concern, given with humor, sometimes anger, and lots of compassion. John loves his wife and boys, his clients, his fellow workers, his friends, and most others not on this list. He belongs to a noble class of people who work quietly, answering the call to serve the poor and weak, and who noisily speak out about the injustice of power systems. These workers, L'Arch assistants, teachers in tough schools, hospice nurses visiting those who are dying, and many others show disinterest in advancing their careers, stockpiling possessions, and empowering themselves. The folks in this layer of soci-

3

ety who provide a buffer between the rich and the poor, the privileged and the marginalized, the strong and the weak, have taken seriously the "preferential option for the poor." They have replaced their *egos* with *Others*. They have distinguished themselves by their answer to the call of the needs of Others.

We should not raise John and his fellow workers too high for honor. They do not, godlike, *create* good work out of some special storage of goodness lodged in their hearts. Rather, they *find* goodness outside themselves in their clients, goodness needing help; and they *respond* with selfless service. They usually do not carry out what ethicists call, "supererogatory acts": those beyond the call of duty. They only do what could be expected of all of us. The call to service addresses not only service providers; it is aimed at us all. Levinas and many others tell us that the call for responsibility to others defines the fundamental feature of the human psyche. John, and others in human services, most people in many ways, and all people in some ways, choose to answer the call.

But the most important thing we must recognize is that none of us *choose* to have the call addressed to us. The call comes to us. The call comes to the human psyche! It comes to each of us from the outside, from the Other, from the inherent dignity, legitimate needs, and essential weakness of our neighbor. We all have our weakness; we all depend on each other; and we all call to each other. Also, we do not *choose* to respond. We choose the manner in which we respond. Turning away is a response. Every kind of response is a response. No one chooses the call, and no one chooses not to respond. No one responds with no response.

Jean, another acquaintance, might be an example of self-corroding cynicism. Expressing a kind of raw pleasure in this activity, Jean frequently throws out these sharp critical observations of the faults of others. She likes to show off her acute observations of their slightest idiosyncracy. She shakes with a kind of delight when she can point out someone's big mistake. Since she also incessantly complains about the weather, the traffic, the government, local cultural habits, and all her neighbors, those who work with her do not take her critical style too seriously. Most of us simply close our ears to her cynicism, having gotten used to her. But we have also become inoculated from frequent injections of cynicism in popular culture nowadays.

Having maneuvered her way into a middle position of authority, Jean blames others when things go badly. She rose to her position of power by convincing those above her that she could do a better job than the former director. But things have gotten worse under her management. While efficiency in the agency suffers and morale fades, she defines herself more and more as the victim. She takes advantage of all the perks of the office and legitimates new ones based on her sense of personal justice for the trouble her supervisors have caused her and their stupidity for not paying attention. However, she does not seem to be happy in this "position of power."

But we should not judge Jean too harshly. Her cynical psyche seems a product of modern advanced society. Jean had all the learning advantages this highly evolved society has to offer. She received degrees in social work and has attended many seminars in management. She learned sophisticated knowledge about how people think and behave, how social structures and processes operate, skills in critical analysis to contrast efficient from inefficient stratagems, and motivational programs to increase productivity. But Jean did not receive in her socialization process an accompanying lesson in modesty and self-questioning. She was designated for early success, trained to move rapidly through the system, and protected from failure and any insights about the paradoxes of power. The educational system, the organized social structure, and the enticements to success by marketing have all paradoxically sabotaged her.

PSYCHOLOGY'S CONTRIBUTION TO THE CYNICISM OF MODERN IDEOLOGIES

Rather than blaming Jean, let me briefly outline what has been the anticipated outcomes of modernity, how the expectations have been fulfilled, and how modernity's success has paradoxically produced such cynicism. Hopefully, this brief and simple description will help to build the case for questioning modern psychology's contribution to our cynical nihilism. I will organize my outline around the three traditional psychological levels: the cognitive, behavioral, and affective styles.

Cognitive enlightenment and our release from ignorance have been the crowning achievement of modernity. Within the cognitive realm, both the natural and human sciences have exploded in knowledge over the last 300 years, accelerating each century and decade the production of methods, theories, facts, and their resultant "truths." Moreover, scientific knowledge has been widely dispersed, offered to most contemporary citizens through schools and the media. While there are still many of us naive about physics, chemistry, biology, and other modern sciences, all have become at least casual students of human behavior and many claim to be rather good practical psychologists, astute observers of political activity, and skilled micro-managers of at least our own micro-economic systems. The knowledge gained by the human sciences has been commercialized and made available to anyone connected and interested. We consider ourselves perceptive of the intentions and motives of others, and especially of ourselves. This modern knowledge gives us confidence in judging people in our daily lives, planning courses of action, and enjoying our self-confident sophistication in figuring out the meanings of people.

Behavioral efficiency in the actions of machines in the physical realm has helped accomplish our advancement in knowledge about the nature of things. Within the human realm, efficiency in the management of both individual and social actions allows us to smooth out our organizational systems to accomplish highly productive work. People can be trained to do amazingly complicated tasks to become highly effective workers. Mishaps are called mistakes; we expect efficiency if proper techniques are applied. Just as ignorance is inexcusable, so failure due to lack of skill is unacceptable. Where only effort is needed in the use of available application, success is open to everyone. With the refinement of techniques in psychology and personal management for self-improvement and organizational management, modernity has apparently reduced the likelihood of failure.

Finally, *affective enjoyment* of available consumer products has increased to create a comfortable lifestyle for the majority of citizens of the locales of modernity. Within the affective realm, both the accumulation of consumer products and the easy access to entertainment provide nearly instant gratification. With the production and distribution of so much *stuff* and so many *happenings*, we expect every modern citizen can live a life of pleasure like never before. With the advancement of medicine to rid us of pain and machines to replace work, discomfort should be on its way out. All this was anticipated and hoped for with the explosion of knowledge in modern science, the refinement of technology, and the production and market distribution of consumer products.

As we near the end of this extraordinarily productive twentieth century we have found, however, that individual and social *understanding, success*, and *happiness* have not grown like our *science, technology*, and *consumer products* had promised. The mythologies of mastery, progress, and freedom from the hard knocks of a primitive world are in doubt. Postmodern cynicism has accelerated in the last fifty years. This half of the century has seen disillusionment and fear. The last ten years has seen an explosion of signs of cynical despair. Our present cynicism is not simply arrogance, abusive manipulation of others, and self-indulgence. We have always had those problems. Our cynicism is the intertwining of arrogance, manipulation, and indulgence with the deflating of the great expectations of modernity. Rather than getting better, things often seem to be getting worse.

Modern *enlightenment* has frequently turned into postmodern criticism of official knowledge and institutional structures, and deep distrust of most of our fellow citizens. At the cognitive level, our postmodern fears of not knowing what we suspect others know and hide are being fed by ideologies of suspicion. Enlightened demagogues spread their comprehensive and certain explanations of why things are going so badly. Religious, political, economic, and psychological theories calculated to appeal to our vested interests are being offered through sophisticated marketing techniques, mostly over television. These *ideologies* provide us justification for cleansing ourselves of any accountability for problems and criticizing the ignorance, hypocrisy, and culpability of those in charge.

Modern *efficiency* has turned into postmodern manipulation of the system. At the behavioral level, our postmodern fear of failure motivates compulsive control of our immediate environment. We have skillful techniques to manipulate the mechanisms of social control: we learn how to make the system individually work for us. We justify taking advantage of others and the system within the accepted practices of competition. Postmodern cynicism assumes no limits to the ego beyond those put in place by other competitors through their skillful manipulation of the system.

Modern *enjoyment* has turned into postmodern addiction to short-term pleasure at the cost of long-term happiness. At the affective level, our postmodern fear of suffering motivates our driven consumption to indulge instant gratification, turning luxuries into conveniences and finally into necessities. We justify the unjust distribution of goods and painful poverty, the depletion of natural resources and damage to the environment, all under the conviction of the ideologies of individualism that aim toward personal, even if isolated, satisfaction. If I correctly hear the many social critics, especially the political challengers who insist that the incumbents are letting society go to hell in a hand-basket, then all the great advantages of modernity have only turned out to sabotage us.

Let me return to Jean. I have picked out those qualities that allow me to use her as an example of a contemporary cynic. This is unfair. She is more than these qualities. She most frequently works hard trying to make things run smoothly in her agency. In face-to-face situations she is usually kind and considerate of others. I have also picked out those qualities of John that allow me to use him as an example of a contemporary person of responsibility. This is also unfair. He is more than these qualities. He stubbornly holds on to ideals even in the face of failure, loses his temper and criticizes bureaucrats for bungling the paper work on some of his clients, and indulges some habits not good for his health. John's generosity is not purely disinterested. He gets egoistic satisfaction out of helping his clients. John is not perfect. He is human like us all.

Furthermore, I cannot judge Jean too harshly. I find myself not terribly unlike her. Those paragraphs I included just above criticizing science, technology, and the distribution of consumer products are quite cynical. We have all inherited this postmodern style of egocentric cynicism. But as Sloterdijk says, we are unhappy with our cynicism. We long for the simplicity, humility, and patient compassion for each other that would get us closer to an idealized existence. I have no basis to be arrogantly critical of others. I have no justification to be selfishly manipulative of others. I have no right to deny others their needed goods in the process for my indulgent consumption.

The history of the development of the modern era is complex. I wish to attend only to the contribution of psychology to our modern cynicism. While modernity has appropriated psychology's ideological justification for self-interest, we inhabitants are haunted by the faces of Others calling us out of ourselves to honor, respect, and serve them because of their inherent dignity and need.

When I do my own phenomenological reflection on being human, I must be *kynical* of my own self-righteousness because I directly experience that I have no choice in being called to responsibility. Responsibility is assigned me independently of my abilities, my occupational or familial role, even independently of my generosity. I am defined as a human person commanded to be responsible. I sometimes self-righteously try to convince myself and others that I have nobly chosen to be a servant of the needy, but this is my foolishly arrogant ego asserting itself. Authentic service is called, not self-chosen for its own glory.

Cynically, many would say that I do have a choice, and my freedom to choose my own rights should take priority over any needs of others. Cynicism says that John's choices fulfill his own need to be a caretaker, that his service to others arises out of motives of self-interest. But this critical judgment represents a distortion of the social, psychological, and spiritual basis for his self-sacrificing and other-dedicated work. During much of John's day, his psyche resides in and dedicates itself to others, specific others with hurting bodies and anxious souls, not abstract others. Any psychology that interprets John's commitment to others as nothing more than the satisfaction of his own personal needs has founded itself on a narrow cynicism. That kind of restricted cynical interpretation of John represents perhaps a defensive accusation justifying the accuser's own selfishness or, perhaps, a vested ideology. Or it is simply vicious. But most likely this cynicism and its judgments arise out of a culturally based psychology, derived from an *enlightened* scientism that reduces human behavior to natural forces stimulated by an individual need like hunger, or from an even more *enlightened* and galloping *humanism*, a simplistic liberalism that exaggerates individual autonomy.

Psychology has a difficult time describing human experience and behavior other than as events of an ego-centered being solely concerned with itself: either an ego forced by biological and instinctual causes, similar to plants and animals, or a willing ego empowering itself for personal self-esteem. Psychology seems unable to make sense of the stories of genuine *radical altruism*. *Radical altruism is an anomaly that does not fit psychology's fundamental paradigm.*

Although researchers have been studying the psychology of helping and altruism for decades (such as Batson, 1991; R. B. Cialdini et al., 1987; J. F. Dovidio et al.,1990; J. A. Piliavin and H. W. Charng, 1990, to name only a few important representatives), their approach is still based on what Levinas calls fundamental *egology*. Their definitions of altruism are not close to Levinas's understanding of radical altruism. In its science and practice, psychology seems stuck in the paradigm of psychological egology. Whether described as determined or as personally free, the self or ego is the center of the self.

On the other hand, many people learn their home-grown psychology in traditions that make sense out of the paradoxes that placed the ego outside itself, in others. Such paradoxes include notions like "the loss of self in the service of others as the way to gain self," "life coming out of suffering and death to the ego," "weakness revealing strength," and "the needs of others calling each of us out of our selfish selves to help."

As a psychologist, I have been baffled by the effort of much of my profession, in both its research and practice, to make us better able to deny those events of weakness that *happen* to us as mythically valued only to serve the powerful. Most of the self-help texts, according to Gary Greenberg in *The Self on the Shelf* (1994), urge us to define whatever desire we have to help others purely for the sake of others as "disordered and needing recovery." Self-development manuals offer exercises to practice skills to empower oneself for the competitive worldly arenas. Psychology today seems to urge us to orient and justify all our action as efforts to be responsible only for Number One. While people are committed to others (e.g., people like John sacrificing their own comfort to help others), psychology has a thin theoretical basis to understand their altruism.

The challenge to egocentric psychology that I hope to spell out in these pages is not, however, inspired by some pious religious idea or exclusively by Levinas's philosophy. When we look at secular literature, we find it filled with the ironies of both the self-sabotage of egoism and the admiration and honor given to self-sacrificing humble service. These paradoxes have been revealed over and over in literature and history. At least since Homer's *Iliad*, 3,000 years ago, the foolishness of egoic war, arrogance, manipulation, and greed, as well as the honor given for self-sacrifice for the powerless, have been the consistent stories of humankind. The tragic flaw of power weakening itself, and the comedic recognition of the power of the weak because of their weakness, was described 2,300 years ago by Aristotle as the essence of drama and the human psyche. Yet contemporary psychology has still not grasped these paradoxes as central to the human condition. Psychology's choice to model itself after the causal and positivistic thinking of the natural sciences, and after the micro-political thinking of individuals in constant competition for what they decided were limited resources to satisfy private needs, has kept psychology from understanding the paradoxes of the weakness of power and the power of weakness.

PSYCHOLOGY: A PSUKHOLOGY AS WELL AS AN EGOLOGY

One of my theses is that most psychology today, certainly the kind influencing much of popular culture, attends exclusively to the study of the *ego*. The *psyche* of modern psychology is the *ego* establishing itself in the center of the individual personality, constructing its own identity, manipulating its environment to feed its needs, and enjoying the pleasure of satisfying those needs. This is certainly a legitimate science of much of human behavior. But it is badly truncated and wrongly named. It cannot understand authentic giving, that is, *radical altruism*. Modern psychology is not the study of the human psyche's ability to transcend its needs to find a deeper desire. Inspired by Emmanuel Levinas, I suggest we call the science of the ego, *egology*.

Humans are more than isolated egos. The word *psyche* was not originally the center of the self, the center of the personality. The Homeric *psyche*, or ψυχη (*psukhe*) originally meant "breath" (*Oxford English Dictionary*, 2nd ed., vol. 12). Homer used this term also to refer to *life, soul*. The *psukhe* was the soul or spirit gradually breathed into and sustained by the life and love of others, by parents, family, tribe, by those for whom the *psukhe* was to be responsible, ultimately by the Spirit of the universe. A reflective phenomenology can still justify this ancient definition. Others *inspire* this *spirit* into the self. The word "inspire" means "to breath into" another. This ancient *psukhe* did not give birth to itself and direct its effort toward itself, as we find explained in contemporary *egology*. The *psukhe* was a gift from others. Only later, did "psyche" come to mean the center of the private personality. In the story of Western thought and practice, we have altered the meaning of the word "psyche" to justify our ideologies of individualism and self-reliance, the self-sufficiency of self-creation and thereby our self-directed indulgence. This book will try to retrieve the notion of the *psukhe* as the *soul* generated by *others-breathing-into-the-self*, and, passively received, the authentic self is actively called to be a *self-breathing-into-others-for-others*.

On the one hand, I will use the term "egology" for the study of the ego establishing its identity, empowering this identity, avoiding weakness, finding its potential, and focusing on self-development. This ego thinks, acts, and feels as a part of nature (physical, social, what we've called "psychological" nature), where energies compete for control, where power is power and weakness is weakness.

On the other hand, I will use the name *psukhology* to urge the reader to pause, to question the dominant paradigm, to redefine the notion of *psychology*. This *psukhology* is the study of the self's having its identity inspired by others, animated by others, empowered by others, discovering the paradox of the weakness of power and the power of weakness to establish its fundamental identity of responsibility *to-and-for-others*. Psychology should be the study of both the *ego* and the *psukhe*, not reducing one concept to the other, but respecting the real distinction between them, and giving a priority to the *psukhe*'s responsibility for others over the ego's ego-centered obsessions, compulsions, and addictions .

The word *responsibility* is used differently by different people especially during the last few congressional sessions and national elections. Gabriel Moran points out in his recent book, *A Grammar of Responsibility*, that some people use the word to mean that each person should be responsible for themselves, and no one else should be held responsible for them. Others use the word to mean that society should be responsible for those who cannot provide for their own needs. I do not intend to get into this debate. In chapter 2 I will show how Levinas offers the radical definition of *responsibility* as the inherent investment of freedom into the self by others to be used for the sake of others. He is fond of quoting (1982/1985, p. 100) the sentence of Dostoyevsky from *The Brothers Karamazov*, "We are all responsible for all and for all men and before all, and I more than all the others" (Dostoyevsky, p. 264). Levinas explains what he means by quoting this extraordinary sentence.

> This is not owing to such or such a guilt which is really mine, or to offences that I would have committed; but because I am responsible for a total responsibility, which answers for all the others and for all in the others, even for their reponsibility. The I always has one responsibility *more* than all the others. (1982/1985, pp. 98–99)

I will try to unpack this claim of Levinas in chapter 2.

This distinction between the *ego* responsible for itself and the *psukhe* responsible for others is not meant to divide classes of people, to separate out altruists from egoists, or to self-righteously judge between good and bad people. All of us exercise selfish ego functions, and all of us are responsible psukhes. The psychological nature of *responsibility*, basically absent from descriptions of contemporary psychology, inspired this work because of its conspicuous absence.

REFLECTION ON SOCIAL PROBLEMS SHOWS THE PARADOXICAL

One source of my thinking about the anomaly of psychology was in confronting social problems that individual psychology seemed unable to address. Although not formally trained as a social psychologist, my involvement and frustrations in social and political activity, and my observation of the growth of cynicism in myself and others, urged me to see psychology as part of the problem rather than part of the solution. Being introduced to Levinas's philosophy of responsibility made clearer the call for a paradigm shift.

While I reconfirm my point that the world is not made up of two kinds of people, good and bad, I can conveniently distinguish between an egology and psukhology by first acknowledging the obvious truth that the powerful possess and enjoy their power, while the weak suffer their weakness. We notice, however, that powerful people frequently sabotage their own power, and the very weakness of the weak has a power over us. No one, neither the powerful nor the weak, disputes the truth of the power of the powerful. Some powerful people may be uncomfortable with their power, and some weak quite comfortable in their weakness. But the fact that power is powerful and weakness is weak is obvious to all: power empowers, supports, perpetuates, frees its holders; weakness, however, weakens, burdens, limits, even kills those who suffer from it.

Common are the arguments about whether the power of the powerful weakens the weak or whether the weakness of the weak brings on their own suffering. However, no one arbitrarily chooses between these two as lifestyles. In modernism, we assume a common understanding that people choose, defend, and justify their power, and avoid, escape, or excuse their weakness. If people choose weakness, it is for a strange and suspect purpose. The logic of this understanding seems indisputable.

Similarly, to justify their power, the powerful often claim personal qualities of talent and initiative and blame the weak for their own inadequacies and laziness. The weak sometimes justly accuse the powerful, and unjustly excuse their weakness by blaming others. Ideologies of justification on both sides have become highly sophisticated. These claims and accusations, although not the issue of this book, point to the insight that power and weakness are not simply opposites.

With only a slight tilt of our attention toward a deeper focus beyond the obvious, we notice that the weakness of a weak individual holds extraordinary power over us; for example, the vulnerable child commands the attention and protection of those around her. Likewise the power of the powerful forms the foundation of their own kind of vulnerability; for instance, the demands of the bully sabotage his own force.

I want to articulate in this book the *psukhological* paradoxes of the power of weakness and the weakness of power. This *illogical* (oxymoronic) relationship between power and weakness, found so frequently in the lives and events of powerful and weak persons, underlies the political, economic, familial, and societal ironies, conflicts, and happy surprises of daily life. However, the social, political, and economic twists and turns are not the topic here. My subject is the *psukhologically* enigmatic, ambiguous, and ironic events that plague and enrich our intra- and interpersonal lives.

Some people declare the very definition of power to be "the oppression of the weak." There has always been, and always will be the weak, and there will always be oppressive power. Others say that, yes, this may be so, but the name of this power is *injustice*, and we are obligated to bring dignity back into the lives of both the victimized weak and the oppressing powerful by efforts to more deeply understand the conditions supporting this injustice, and to work for justice, peace, compassion, and the defense of life and rights.

Policies, strategies and practices of social activism against injustice are not the point of this book. This book attends to the *psukhological* paradoxes beneath policies, strategies and practices. Because the best-laid stratagems often backfire in the unforeseen ambiguities of social existence, we need to look deeper into these human paradoxes. Practices succeed in spite of overwhelming odds: Davids beat Goliaths. Oppressive power self-destructs: the ambition of Ceasars inspire conspirators against these tyrants. I ask from these examples what constitutes the psukhological paradoxes that lie below these reversals of the best-laid plans, and the successes of the worst. And how can insights into these paradoxes help the science of psychology?

Is the answer hidden in a mysterious plan of a mysterious God, as some religiously faithful believe? Is it a natural selection too complex for us to have yet deciphered, as some positivists believe? Can we assume that, since all humans are created equal, those who design and profit from the suffering of others contribute to an imbalance, and, in a final reckoning, either by divine intervention or natural selection, power will become weak, and weakness will become powerful? Is this paradox explainable by a sacred or secular calculus of reciprocity? These are not my questions. I raise them only because I think much cynicism develops because many people have put their hopes in these religious and mechanistic *ideological* explanations.

Independently of theological, sociological, or philosophical doctrines and disputations, the weak still struggle with their lives against powerful forces. They suffer their wants and insecurity, and anxiety and resignation to even worse suffering. Meanwhile, the powerful may suffer their own anxiety over the tenuousness of their condition and search for always more comfort and a more secure security, while enjoying their privilege.

STATEMENT OF THE PARADOX

To the question, What are the paradoxes of power and weakness? the response is: *power can be the very basis of power's weakness as well as its power; and weakness, still weak, can be the power of the weak.* At the foundation of both the individual and social struggles of weakness against power and power against weakness, we find these *unnatural paradoxes*: power nurtures its own weakness, and weakness possesses its source of power in that weakness.

This reality, however common, must be called *unnatural*, because it does not follow the laws of nature. It is unreasonable because it does not follow the dictates of reason. It is a *para-* ("beyond") + *-dox* ("opinion, teaching, doctrine"). It goes beyond our understanding that is based on that which we ordinarily expect. It defies the logical; it is *psukhe-logical*. The *psukhe* is not a piece of nature. Its unnatural nature is paradoxical.

For the focused attention to the paradoxical, I again suggest the name, both difficult to spell and pronounce, *psukhology*, to deliberately remind readers to resist the effort to reduce the study of the paradoxical to the study of some natural law of organic and/or behavioral forces within the individual person: the dispositions, the habits, the traits, and the personality styles studied by the modern science of *egology*. My effort is to remind the reader that the *psyche*, besides being an *ego*, is a *psukhe*; it is the soul gradually breathed into the person and continuously nourishing its life of responsibility with the breath of the souls of others. Others inspire, breathe into, the self responsible ways of relating back to proximate and distant others: parents, ancestors, descendants, contemporaries, neighbors, loved ones, even enemies, whoever touches the self. This fundamental paradox of the origin of the humaneness of the human reveals the *psukhe-logical.* Contrarily, the facts of egology are not paradoxical; they are logical, natural, linearly causal.

Being unnatural, the paradox of the weakness of power cannot be made *doxical* (sensical) by reducing it to a simple conflict between two defined forces, one strong and one frail. This paradox cannot be read simply as an abstract lesson from the mythical and historical stories of the battles between a *power* that has lost its might and loses the struggle against a *weakness* that has surprisingly increased its strength. The weakness of the powerful is not the challenge from another power; the weakness of the powerful lies in their own power. The powerful hold on to their power, and it is precisely this egoistic holding of power that makes them vulnerable to weakness. Tyrants, perhaps originally motivated for the good of the people, gradually protect power for the sake of power, and are thereby toppled because they lose the loyalty of their people.

Likewise, the power of the weak is not the gaining of some new power. The weak are still weak, but their weakness is the source of their power. The blind person at the street corner stops traffic because of her or his lack of sight. It is weakness that powerfully stops traffic. These paradoxes reveal that the powerful, as powerful, are weak, and the weak, by their weakness, are powerful.

Analogously, the paradox cannot be reduced to the simple feature of a complex social distribution in which everyone has a portion of power and their share of weakness. Although many self-improvement books and programs claim that the only thing each person must do is look within his or her own weakness to find the natural source of power, to further empower that source, and use it in the competitive situations of life. Their simple prescription, in part at least, misses the point.

This book will not offer a self-development manual instructing how to use one's weakness to gain power over others. Although chapter 3 on power, and chapter 4 on weakness, mimic a bit the self-improvement books, the paradox we will look at in chapters 5 and 6 lies deeper in the human psyche and its social relations. *It is the very power of the powerful that is the source of their weakness, and the very weakness of the weak that is the source of their power.* It is the task of these pages to describe the psukhological features of this double-edged paradox.

Many books about the economic and political events of society articulate and exemplify the negative features of the sharp edge of power. I will let the economist describe the poverty of the affluent. I will leave the political scientist to point out the vulnerability of tyrants and revolutionaries. The educator-epistemologist can describe better than I the foolishness of narrow intellectual, logical, and rational minds. And especially will I let the biblical exegete spell out the gospel meaning of the threats of woe to the powerful: "Woe to you rich . . . , woe to you who are now filled . . . , woe to you when all speak well of you . . . , for you shall be humbled."

I will also leave it to specialized experts to describe the other side of the paradox found in the riches of the unencumbered life of voluntary poverty, the political force of the gathered disenfranchised, the profound wisdom of the simple uneducated, and the blessedness of the weak. In these and other examples of social ironies we find the psukhological paradox of the power of weakness and the weakness of power.

This book also does not focus on what psychologists call the "passive-aggressive" pattern or disposition. Feigning weakness to manipulate others implies that the one so acting knows, at some level, the paradox of the power of weakness, and that this paradox could work for him or her. Yet the actual use of this deception implies that this fraudulent sufferer does not know that, as only a trick, this power itself is ultimately weak; or, that sham weakness is a self-destructive power, a gamble that the perpetrator's deception won't be found out and boomerang back to weaken him or her. We do want to ask, however, what it is that the passive-aggressive knows, at least in an unreflective way, if not in reflective calculation.

We especially want to ask: What is it about weakness that so moves others to lend their power? and what is it about power that makes it so likely to self-sabotage?

THE PARADOX OF THE POWER OF WEAKNESS

Let me expand the example of the weak child. If most of us were to find an infant left lying in a public place vulnerable to harm by natural or human forces, we would unhesitatingly lend our power of protection. We would pick the child up, hold her or him, and search for the parent or guardian. We would likely do whatever was needed to provide the power the child lacked. If the child was suffering and hungry, we would deny our own comfort to get food, spending money and time to support her or him in this weakness. The weak infant possesses paradoxical power.

A less obvious example is the adult found lying in a similar fragile position and place, helpless in a potentially harmful situation. We make a quick and uncertain decision about whether the person is potentially strong enough to get back into safety, or if the person's weakness can only be helped by our intervention. Most people ask if the person needs help.

The difficult examples are of people who seem to have placed themselves in their weakened state by their own power. An adult lying in a public place vulnerable to the same harm, but presumably there by previous choices, like drinking too much alcohol, does not inspire all of us to help. When weakness is obviously self-imposed, many of us do not lend power to help out. Perhaps we conclude that giving help would only increase the dependency of the weak, and support their self-destructive behavior. The popular term *dependency* is certainly legitimate in many cases. Aid adds to weakness, we often conclude. We judge that the irresponsible are not the un-responsible, and that those who are presently weak have the possibility and responsibility to eventually get out of their suffering. We often judge that this kind of irresponsibility deserves the pain of weakness, and that the only hope for those in this condition lies in their desire to escape from this punishment. This desire will be the incentive to freely will themselves back into personal power with self-help.

Other bystanders, however, judge that the weak, even if it seems they are responsible for their own weakness, still need help. Their decision to help is likely based on a few philosophical assumptions, to be more fully described in chapter 2. The first assumption behind helping another is that an observer cannot fully know that another is solely responsible for her or his own weakened condition: *the Other is beyond comprehensive understanding.* The opposite assumption is shaky: since the person made choices that got him or her there, he or she can make new choices to get out. A second assumption supporting helping is that we all have responsibility, by our human existence, for each other, both in how we get into places of vulnerability and how we get out: *the Other's weakness calls us, even commands us, to be responsible.* And finally, this judgment of the call to respond carries a third, very frustrating assumption that embodies the paradoxical, that is, that although we are able to help, although we have within us the capability, the power to reduce another's suffering, yet our help cannot reduce them and their weakness to the object of our power: *the Other is infinitely nearby commanding help, and infinitely distant, always exceeding our total understanding and our power to control.*

The insightful Bishop Kenneth Untener of Saginaw, in his request that diocesan personnel spend three months attending to the impact diocesan decisions would have on the poor, asked them to consider, "How shall what we are doing here affect or involve the poor?" He arrived at a list of insights ("The Decree to Discuss the Poor: What Was Learned?" *Origins*, August 1991) that embody these previously stated philosophical assumptions.

> (1) We tend to forget the poor poor. (2) The poor are often invisible. (3) The biggest problems are raised by the *undeserving* poor: help them help themselves; address the deeper conditions before you blame; and err on the side of largesse. (4) If you try to help the poor, you will sometimes get taken. (5) Helping the poor is not always a pleasant experience. (6) Food baskets at

Thanksgiving, toys at Christmas are good as far as they go, but they don't go very far. (7) Sometimes the poor are overwhelmed into inaction. (8) The poor also help the poor. (p. 164–66).

He points out that when we get too caught up in distinguishing the *deserving* from the *undeserving*, we get into an endless rationalizing conflict. Both the deserving and the undeserving suffer. Their suffering calls out to us to help. It does not call for our judgment about their previous free choices and therefore deservedness. Admittedly, everyone's suffering does not call us to give the same response, but it does call us, just the same.

Over and above their philosophical or political differences, those partisans who lean toward positions and policies for individual responsibility and power, and those who stress communitarian responsibility and power, hear or read with disgust about people who callously neglect the suffering of others, those who protect their own precious power solely for themselves and do not lend it to the weak. Both individualists and communitarians consider this kind of selfishness a weakness in character. Neither individualism nor communitarianism defends egocentric individualism that turns away from others' neediness.

Elie Weisel, like Jean Vanier, speaks for all of us.

In the face of suffering, one has no right to turn away, not to see. In the face of injustice, one may not look the other way. When someone suffers, and it is not you, he comes first. His very suffering gives him priority.

We are especially shocked and outraged by those who deliberately take advantage of others' weaknesses and psychologically, physically, or sexually abuse them. We tolerate, sometimes admire, and sometimes even honor attacks against the powerful. We condemn, however, violence against the weak, the widow, the orphan, the destitute. Fellow inmates show bank robbers respect, but brutalize convicted child molesters.

Yet the occasions when people take advantage of the weak and use power to worsen the defenseless suffering of others are so common that many social scientists and their philosophies would argue that this claimed *paradox of the power of weakness* is just another attempt to support a moral myth. It is not really a characteristic of the human condition. This claimed paradox is an idealistic vision of justice, perhaps for rhetorical and partisan ideology. Given the state of modern theoretical, and often practical ethics (MacIntyre, 1981; Cushman, 1990), the suspicion is not surprising.

QUICK SURVEY OF ETHICAL THEORIES

In contrast to the radical alterocentrism offered by Levinas, the following quick review from Rachels (1993) of the major ethical theories shows how they tend to be ego-centered and self-sabotaging. An ethical theory like that of Levinas that is centered in the rights of others exposes its fragility when it confronts the "muscular ethical theories centered in the ego," to quote my son, Matthew. The ethical philosophies centered in the ego exemplify the power of power and betray their power by their own power.

Many contemporary *enlightened* observers hold a dim and cynical view of human goodness and acts of altruism as anything other than self-interest. Their theories tend to be either cultural relativism (right and wrong are the products of the customs of any particular culture) or psychological relativism (*right* and *wrong* are the products of the psychological choices of the private individual).

Another theory, moral contractualism, claims that neighbors form implicit and often explicit contracts to avoid violating each other because they do not want those others (or her brothers) to come back for violent revenge.

Utilitarianism claims that together and alone, people only act to maximize happiness: "The greatest happiness for the greatest number." Peace makes them happy, and violence makes them unhappy. Nonviolence is useful; it lets people get on with their lives of happiness.

These ethical theories (relativism, contractualism, and utilitarianism) that guide many psychologists, sociologists, economists, and political scientists are essentially egologies. Recognizing the shallowness of these approaches, Neo-Kantianism offers an ethical theory in contrast to the self-interest theories. Emmanuel Kant claimed that the origin of ethics lies in the ability of *reason* to arrive at moral requirements. Each of us goes through this explicit or implicit reasoning, "Since I would want others to never lie or kill me, I can claim their prohibitions to be universal principles, applying to everyone." These universally applicable principles are called by Kant "categorical imperatives" and are distinguished from "hypothetical imperatives." On the one hand, hypothetical imperatives are those actions we ought to do given the hypothesis that we want a certain result, for example, to learn to drive a car one ought to practice driving; if one does not want to learn driving, practice is not imperative. Categorical imperatives, on the other hand, are commanded of everyone. Reason, a universal ability of all human selves, has the power to keep emotions and personal motives from distorting our categorical imperatives. Therefore everyone should have a sense of duty. Reason self-legislates in the realm of morality.

Modern social scientists, however, tend to hold that the Kantian belief in a morality based on the power of reason has been undermined by depth psychology, which shows that primitive narcissistic desires contaminate the very core of reason itself. They say our parents have introjected into our conscience whatever morality we seem to possess. Sociobiologists, equally suspicious of reason, claim we are genetically inclined either to violence or to care, or to a mixture. These attacks on Kant's theory of the supremacy of reason still claim that the force for or against moral action originates within the person. Responsibility begins in either the determined or the autonomous ego, not in the call to us originating from the needs of others; ethics begins in the self rather than from the Other.

Some ethicists are returning to a sort of Aristotelian focus on the notions of virtue and of natural right action. But the natural law theory centered in personality virtues is also based on the assumption that the ego is the center and origin of ethical behavior. With sufficient help from parents and other models each person will cultivate virtues and grow into a responsible citizen. Goodness is the quality of virtues and virtues are properties of the ego.

Natural law, contractualism, utilitarianism, and Kantian rationalism are all *egologies.* Their first assumption is that the origin of moral behavior is centered in the ego self-initiating its good intentions and actions.

The radical alternative to egoistic theories of ethics points out that the neediness[1] and worthiness of others, calling us to responsibility *prior* to our reason, *beyond* our individual desire for happiness, *before* forming any contract with others, generates the ethical command. This alternative is a radical *alterocentrism.* It calls for a radical *alterology*, a radical *psukhology.* It can be described as *radical altruism.*

Truly this call to be responsible and this paradox of the power of the weakness of the Other are not physical or biological laws of nature, nor are they certainly sociological or psychological laws. Human nature tends to be egocentric, cynically ignoring conscience, claiming the priority of *personal freedom* over *responsibility-by-and-for-Others.* Being responsible goes against nature. Ethics founded on the paradox of the power of the weakness of others over us, and the weakness of our egoistic power is not natural. Ethics is beyond nature. Ethical behavior transcends the ego's natural jostling with others for its place in the sun. A psukhology inspired

---

1. The terms *neediness* and *needy* are not used here with any pejorative meaning. This is the nature of the human: to have needs.

by the ethical behavior toward the neediness of others would have to define the human as more than an object of nature responding to the forces of nature.

Claiming that the laws of nature do not generate ethical behavior is not a claim that ethical behavior is rare. Humans relatively consistently respond with responsibility toward their fellow humans. The secret Vanier speaks of is not, as he points out, so secret to so many. He ironically calls it a "secret." Although responsibility is not a law of nature, responsible behavior is an evident, empirical fact. People help out those in need. We might be tempted to claim that there is a quasi-habit to help, calculable by an inverse relation between the weakness of the needy person and the paradoxical power it has over us: the greater the weakness, the more likely we are to lend our power. The depth of the other's weakness determines the level of our help. For example, the younger the child, the more care it commands. The more the other's poverty seems to flow from conditions other than laziness, from conditions they could not help, the more likely we are to give generously. When another's pathology is seen more as an affliction than a result of poorly chosen behavior, the more sacrifices we willingly make to relieve it.

The power of the weak is that the person's weakness calls us to respond generously. When the call goes out to us we obviously have our individualized liberty either to give or to turn away from this call of the weak. We have the power, in the form of freedom, to respond either with help, or with selfishness, even viciousness. But we do *not* have the freedom to choose whether or not we are called. The call has its source outside of us coming from the weakness of the weak. The power of the weak is the Other's neediness. It commands us to respond to weakness.

When Elie Weisel says "one has no right . . . one may not look the other way . . . " he is saying that the *I* is singled out, I am assigned, I am the *one* appointed. I can't pass responsibility on. When I look, my very seeing designates me as more than a watcher. My exposure to the Other commands me to do more than see: I am assigned to open the eyes of my eyes and to serve the Other in her or his weakness. For each of us, signification comes before freedom. Being assigned responsibility comes before any autonomous will to respond. The Other's call signifies me before I am free to answer the call in my own chosen way. My election by others to be responsible precedes and is therefore independent of my capabilities and opportunities to be generous or selfish. Responsibility is universally commanded, even though it appears to be disregarded by so many of us protecting our precious individual freedom. I cannot use others' irresponsibility to justify my own. Belief in the *primacy of individual freedom* over the *primacy of responsibility* is an idealistic myth used to legitimate the

practices of an ego-esteeming culture supported by an ideological infra-
structure. Against this myth, we are called to be countercultural. Each of
us is called, but I can only speak for myself. *I am appointed. I am ordained. I
am named.*

Another weakness (briefly implied above in the statement of the
philosophical assumption about simultaneous *nearness* and *distance*)
reveals itself in this relation between those who call and those called: *the
power of those called can never resolve the weakness of the weak.* I can help out; I
can reduce the pain; I can give access to my own and other sources of
power. But perhaps my greatness psychological weakness is in my self-
delusions that I can fully understand another's condition, that I can totally
relieve another's neediness, that I have the power to create fulfillment in
another. An authentic ethical response does not justify self-righteousness.
The self neither initiates nor completes any ethical action. I am simply and
always commanded. Being appointed does not give me dignity deserving
honor; it only gives me responsibility.

This ambiguity, on the one hand, of the undeniable call, and, on the
other, the impossibility of completing what is asked of me is paradoxical:
the Other is both always and everywhere *proximate*, close to me (calling
me before I can choose to respond, even calling me before her or his immediate needs call me), and yet always and everywhere *distant* (far from me,
beyond the reach of my efforts to reduce her or him to an object of my generous and noble efforts in answering her or his call).

The otherness of the Other, her or his radical independence, is always
the otherness of that person. The Other's otherness is not a limitation in
me, an ignorance, a physical distance. The origin of her or his otherness is
from their absolute worthiness. No one is a thing reducible to an object of
my knowing, my controlling its conditions. All humans, even those
whose actions are deserving of punishment and denial of some rights, are
beings with a source of dignity of their own; each is ultimately not within
my context, but is an independent nobility. Yet each is always there beside
me, commanding responsibility of me. The dignity of the Other's weakness (worthy to call) places her or him beyond my power (impotent to
reduce). The frustration of the inadequacy of my generous response can
humble me more than the admission of my selfish responses.

THE PARADOX OF THE WEAKNESS OF POWER

The other side of this same paradox offers a mirror image of the power of
weakness: the powerful indeed have power, but this power is the source
of their weakness. Although the powerful often attract admiration and

imitation, and, by their promise for our gain, even seduce us to suffer the abuse of their power, there is a psychological tendency to be suspicious and repulsed by the claims of self-initiated and self-directed power. We sometimes align ourselves with the powerful against the weak in pursuit of our own ego-centered power. But the power of the powerful does not force our allegiance. We collaborate with power, and then at times, defensively rationalize our weakness to pursue power. We know power serves our needs, but we also know that it can whip back, strike us, and make us weak. The seduction of power is an illusion, but a seduction none the less.

When we are psychologically captured and driven by our own power, we know that our bondage is, first, our addiction to the sweet taste of power itself; second, our addiction to the stuff that power can purchase; third, our habitual blindness to the needs of others; and, finally, our fear of losing the power to exercise more power. Obsessive fear, compulsive needs, and sensory indulgence are the weaknesses of power. Self-perpetuating needs and fear of others' taking our power drive us into ourselves and away from others. The power of power can be self-destructive. It tends to burrow into and cling to the heart, rather than expose itself to the needy claims of others. Although I know this by watching others corrupted by power, I most clearly know this paradox of the weakness of power from my own self-corroding tendencies.

Just as the weakness of the weak calls me to help the weak, so does their weakness call me to challenge powerful others to serve the weak. Although, I am not free in being called to challenge the power of powerful others, I am free in the way I respond. I can be seduced by power, or I can oppose it. But it is the weakness of the weak that calls me to challenge power. Conscience is con- ("together with") + -scire ("to know"). Conscience is not a private whisper; it is knowing together, knowing that others know that we know. Not only do we "have no right to turn away" from the suffering of others, and to lend our power, but we are also called to bear witness to still others for the suffering of the weak.

I was struck several years ago, as I watched on television the great anthropologist Richard Leakey say that if it were only the fittest who survive, this fragile human species would not have come so far with so many weak members. The weak of the species have been powerful in commanding the strong, especially as a community, to protect them. The Darwinian thesis, a thesis that seems to be waning in importance in our biological sciences, but still waxing in our social sciences, especially in psychology, economics, and political science is challenged by the thesis that is beyond any thesis: *ethical responsibility.* Weakness ethically *com-*

mands power, precisely because it is unable to physically *demand* it by force.

THE ITINERARY

I have an obligation to readers to show the roots of most of my insights in the ethical phenomenology of Emmanuel Levinas. I borrow from him much of what I have already written in these first pages, and what I will write in the following chapters. I can only hope that I do not dishonor his extraordinary thinking. His books, mainly *Totality and Infinity*, and *Otherwise than Being: or, Beyond Essence*, make a radical turn from the course of the Greek generated Western philosophy that has provided the paradigm for modern social science. Therefore, part I, chapter 2 will be a non-scholarly but serious attempt to describe the key insights I have received from him.

In part II chapters 3 and 4, I will attempt a phenomenology of power and weakness. The task of phenomenology is to make explicit by the use of rigorous reflection on that which is lived out at the more implicit level. Phenomenology attempts to hold back prejudice and bias, including cultural habits and customs, theoretical and scientific concepts, and even personal styles, in order to reflect on the essence of a phenomenon as clearly as possible, and to describe it in general and understandable terms. This method is not for the exclusive use of those who belong to a modern philosophical tradition called phenomenology. We have a right to expect all social analysts to be unbiased. For example, we could expect any worthy and honest political scientist to describe the structures and processes of political activity (the events of people organized to maintain order through the use of government) without tainting his or her descriptions by advocating partisan ideologies and election techniques (the uses and abuses of political power). The same should be expected of an economist, a sociologist, a psychologist.

However, phenomenology, like other epistemological methods, is vulnerable to subtle self-deception. Reflecters and describers can convince themselves that they are clean of cultural and theoretical prejudice, and yet not recognize a deeper pre-reflective influence. For example, I will begin chapter 3 with the assumption that I could reflect and describe an unbiased phenomenological analysis of the experience of *power*. A phenomenology of personal power should simply make explicit what is assumed to be obvious to the careful reflection of any person. Therefore, I will begin with this assumption of obviousness. My method of reflection will be the simple act of *disclosing* what is commonly known to be known by anyone who looks and thinks about power. Objective thinking assumes the phenomenon is able to be read the same by everyone. My method of description to others of this objective *disclosure* will be *declaring* how power is shown to everyone that it is powerful.

However, given my insight about the paradox of the weakness of power, I know these *disclosures* and *declarations* are susceptible to bias from my position of power attempting to write objectively about power. My method must either not take into account this insight about the paradoxical, or take it into account. My method to describe power *objectively* must be either foolish or ironic. Since I've confessed my insight, I cannot claim naive foolishness. The disclosures and declarations of chapter 3 are given ironically. I will ironically play the role of the "general observer" in his or her voice of the first-person plural pronoun "we," assuming the intersubjective "we" to be more objective than the personal "I," which is suspected of being too subjective. For example, I will disclose and declare, "*We* know what power is. Power is intelligence, it is skill, it is satisfied needs. And we know that our power can accumulate more power." So the use of the "we" is arrogant, I hope ironically arrogant, since I am really only an "I," not having consulted others assumed in the "we," yet assuming they would disclose and declare just as I.

I do not have the space in this book, or the philosophical sophistication, to do an adequate review of the epistemological question of objectivity. When I went to graduate school I learned how Edmund Husserl (1913/1950; 1931/1960), the founder of the school of phenomenology, outlined a philosophy and methodology to achieve *objectivity* in describing the events of human consciousness. Merleau-Ponty (1942/1967; 1945/1962; 1964), Husserl's student, was the biggest influence on me in my 1967–71 graduate studies. But it was Emmanuel Levinas who enlightened me with the insight that even a phenomenological description can embody a subtle prejudice, especially an egological prejudice.

In chapter 4, I will point out that, since weakness is weak, we often attempt to hide our own weakness, or at least excuse it. Yet sometimes we use our weakness to passive-aggressively manipulate others. Therefore, in order to avoid any prejudice about my own weakness, and to strive for objectivity, I will reflect on my observation of others and describe their weakness, rather than use self-reflection. Chapter 4 will be a phenomenological reflection and description of the origin of, and thus accountability for, the *weakness of the weak*. The method will be *exposing* and *accusing*.

However, the method here in chapter 4 must be even more self-consciously, more ironically arrogant than that of chapter 3. Here I will be pretending to assume myself, as describer, free of weakness while finding it in others. The *exposures* and accusations in chapter 4 are still within the egological paradigm. The weakness of others is observed and reflected upon, and then described by me, the righteous observer, in the voice of the first person plural pronoun, almost royal or pontifical, "we," exposing the weakness of the third-person singular pronouns, following her or his introduction as the "person."[2] For example, "we are not so blind that we cannot see that that person is weak, and that she is hurting others and herself." I hope that this openly arrogant methodology helps to expose the problem of *egology*: if I begin from my ego, I inevitably violate the Other.

The reflections and descriptions in this part II, chapters 3 and 4, will have laid the ground for part III, chapters 5 and 6, for the *psukhological paradox* of the weakness of my own power, and the power of the weakness of the Other. The *egological* prejudice only partially revealed in part II, will be more explicitly shown to be *egological* by way of contrast to the psukhological methods in part III. In other words, chapter 3 will have been "macho" without admitting to it at the time: "I know power." I, as describer, will have demonstrated a self-righteous superiority. In chapter 4 I will have been even abusive of the weak in my accusations of the person's weakness, while hiding my abusiveness behind the effort to be objective. But the reader will, I hope, be able to see through my intended irony. My power will show a kind of weakness weaker than the obvious weakness of the person I describe. My bravado in describing (bragging about) my power in chapter 3, and my tendency toward violence in describing (vicious blaming) the weakness of the other in chapter 4, will now be exposed in part III as having been arrogant and vicious. Because I was arrogantly accusing her or him, the neediness of the Other confronts and accuses me of a self-righteous, egocentric violence, a tendency (weakness) to violate her or his fundamental integrity and dignity. In chapter 4, I was more than abusive; I was cynically abusive. I tried to demonstrate my acute perception of the Other's weakness, but was, in fact, unperceptive of my own weakness, my tendency to abuse the person. (I will return to Sloterdyjke's definition of cynicism, "enlightened false consciousness," finally in an Interlude before chapter 7.)

This experience of being confronted by the victim of my methodological accusation and cynicism *exposes* me as violent. This exposure urges me to turn to new phenomenological methods for part III, chapters 5 and 6. The method of reflection is not a method in the sense of a chosen tactic to disclose a phenomenon. The origin of my reflection is in the Other's calling me to admit my ego-centeredness. I am passive to *being exposed*, and to

---

2. This phenomenological *exposing* and *accusing* is distinguished from the research that Habermas says comes out of emancipatory *interests* (J. Haberman, 1972, *Knowledge and Human Interest*). Similarly, this is not the same as the *critical psychology* of de Boer (T. de Boer, 1983, *Foundations of a Critical Psychology*).

being called to responsibly admit it. My method of reflection and description of the paradox of the weakness of power, in chapter 5, will be *being exposed* and *confessing* to the reader my weakness toward violence. I am thrown back upon myself because I myself have been exposed as cynically abusive and am called to be responsible for my egological accusations, having attempted to claim in chapters 3 and 4 unbiased phenomenological reflections and descriptions, but now admitting my hypocrisy. My admissions of exposure are described in my *confessions* in the voice of the exposed first-person singular pronoun "I." "Here I am. I have been exposed. I admit I have abused the Other, and I am sorry."

But the dignity and neediness of the Other does more than expose me, accuse me, and command me to admit and confess. The Other calls me out of my ego-centeredness to transcend my ego-centeredness to responsibly be open to, serve, and sacrifice for the Other. The Other confronts me and calls me to avoid the tendency to use my confession to escape from the presence of her or his proximity by the use of an (egological) self-abdication, a giving up on myself in order to avoid responsibility, or to purify myself by way of self-flagellation. The neediness of the Other has the power to call me not to escape my identity, but to identify myself as responsible to know, serve, and sacrifice for the Other. This confrontation by the face of the Other neither debases nor minimizes my responsibility. It consecrates it, beyond my sanctimonious justification, because I am never the origin of my own responsibility, nor am I ever able to be absolutely successful in my knowledge, service, and sacrifice for the Other. My freedom, even to be responsible, is invested in me by the neediness of the Other. My freedom ought to be used responsibly for the Other. The method of reflection in chapter 6 will be, therefore, *listening to and being touched by the call to responsibility.* The method of description of this paradox of the power of weakness is humbly responding, "Here I am."

I hope to show that the origin of authentic phenomenology to exercise the most trustworthy *epoché*, bracketing prejudice for honest reflection, is from the Other. When I set out from my own ego to objectively reflect and describe my experiences of power and weakness of others, as I do in part II, I am inevitably biased. When my reflection and description of others is drawn out by the command of the Other for me to be honest, which happens when the Other faces me, then I am more likely to be honest than when privately reflecting. The face of the Other calls me to be honest. Certainly, I do not deceive myself into thinking that I cannot lie to another facing me; yet the face of the Other acts as a more commanding source of honesty than my own interest in being honest. Levinas's philosophy, as described in chapter 2, will help make clearer the methodology I intend to use in the book.

In part IV, I begin with a brief Interlude interrupting the progression established to move from the one-on-one dyad to the larger social situation of other Others, of triads, quatrads, multiple others. The extravagant claims of Levinas's *heteronomy* (radical altruism) where the Other has rights over the self, and the *self-skepticism, self-substitution,* and *self-sacrifice* described in chapter 6 seem "too much" for many of my students. I respond to their objections first by defending these idealistic descriptions of holiness by referring to Edith Wyschogrod's *Saints and Postmodernism* (1990). I then refer to Peter Sloterdijk's *Critique of Cynical Reason* (1983/1987) to show how our modern cynicism might conclude that this idealism is "too much." Finally, I justify placing limits on self-skepticism, self-substitution, and self-sacrifice not by reverting back into *egology*, but by Levinas's radical *heteronomy*, referring to Roger Burggraeve's *From Self-Development of Solidarity: An Ethical Reading of Human Desire in its Socio-Political Relevance according to Emmanuel Levinas* (1985).

Finally in chapter 7, other Others make their appearance. The Other who inspires me is not just an isolated Other, but represents other Others: all others. I find myself not only responsible for the proximate Other, but for the distant Other as well, paradoxically pointed to by the presence of the immediately proximate Other. There is never just the Other. There is always a third, a fourth, a hundredth, and so on. We are always a community, and each is responsible for all. The incarnate presence of the Other (always needy: hungry, thirsty, ill, homeless, depressed, anxious, suffering even in affluence and comfort) assigns me as the one responsible for others, and even responsible for the responsibility of other Others: to call others to community responsibility, because I certainly neither can nor should do it all. The organization of society both extends the call to me *from* other Others, more people than I ever meet face to face, to everyone; and society extends my responsibility *through* the help of other Others, more people than I can even imagine, through the institutional structures of society.

This recognition of my responsibility to other Others when the face of the nearby Other confronts me, often challenges my too facile response. I am questioned: How does the face of the Other represent all other humanity? I may see someone on the street and respond as if he represents all of humanity, yet be blind to the needs of this particular person. I tend to objectify this immediate person as "the representative of all humankind." Other times, I am called to an individual Other but lose sight of the face of humanity revealed there. I am so caught up in responding here and now that I forget my responsibility to others perhaps more needy. But then, no one ever promised that community responsibility would be easy.

The method of reflection and description of the paradox of the *power of community* in chapter 7 will be the social exposure of needs and rights, and the *communication* with each other of our *assignments* of academic/political/economic responsibilities to serve needs and respect rights. The method could be called "dialogal phenomenology."[3] The phenomenology of communicating our responsibilities, and assigning these responsibilities to each other will be from a "we," but neither from the objective (arrogant) "we," as in macho chapter 3, nor from the imperial (cynically abusive) "we," as in chapter 4. The reflections and descriptions will not be from the confessing accountable "I" of chapter 5, nor from the individually responsible "I" of chapter 6. The reflections and descriptions will be from a communitarian "we." "We are responsible. How do we do what we need to do?"

Before we do the five phenomenological reflections and descriptions, let us turn the page to chapter 2, and open up some magnificent philosophical insights of Emmanuel Levinas.

---

3. I am deeply indebted to my colleagues here at Seattle University Psychology Department, especially Steen Halling, Michael Leifer, and Jan Rowe, for their pioneering work in developing the method of *dialogal phenomenology* (Leifer, 1986; Halling and Leifer, 1991; Halling, Kunz, and Rowe, 1994).

CHAPTER TWO

An Alternative Paradigm

The Philosophy of Emmanuel Levinas

THE PSUKHE (BREATH, SPIRIT, SOUL) IS THE-OTHER-IN-ME

An extraordinary teacher told me he has for years asked his students to read Graham Greene's novel, *The Power and the Glory*. The power of the powerless characters in this book teach directly the most important lesson of his course. The central character is a "bad" priest, an alcoholic and adulterer. Running from the police, he remembers nostalgically the days when his parishioners doted on him. He admits his self-indulgence, and his cowardice. He suffers the loneliness of hiding and seeks others, yet knows his presence in villages in a Mexican state that oppresses religion puts the peasants in jeopardy. He loves his illegitimate daughter and cannot feel guilty for her existence. Nor can he turn down the request to minister to a murderer, even when he knows it is a trap. He confesses the corruption of his own ego, and gives himself completely to others. Greene did not show the simplicity, humility, and patient compassion of this character in order to exempt the rest of us. Inspired by my teacher's assignment, I still reread this book every few years. The fallible but holy provide us a model. Edith Wyschogrod revives for us, in her book *Saints and Postmodernism* (1990), the value of reading the lives of saints, "those who put themselves totally at the disposal of the Other" (p. xiv), for understanding ethics.

"*The psyche in the soul is the Other in me, a malady of identity*" (Levinas, 1974/1981, p. 69).

What an extraordinary definition of the psyche or psukhe: *the Other in me*! Irrational it may be; but, for Levinas, and for Graham Greene, for innumerable writers of stories about ethical characters, and for the saints who are the models of ethical behavior, this is the essential characteristic of the human: *the essence of the self is to seek the good revealed in others, and, in*

31

this way, the self finds it authenticity working for the sake of others. We could say it either way: *the self finds the Other-in-the-self,* or, *the self finds itself-in-the-Other.* Levinas calls this *heteronomy.* (Although risking the creation of an oxymoronic term, I will use *alterocentrism* in place of his term *heteronomy,* to contrast with the term *egocentrism.*)

To our Western individualistic way of thinking and acting, this *heteronomy* or *alterocentrism* strikes us as too radical, too difficult to swallow. We are too cynical to imagine such an ontologically radical altruism: *finding oneself in the Other while the Other retains her or his absolute otherness.* We tend to find ourselves reducing the Other to something for the self, reducing her or his absolute otherness to fit the self. This reduction of the distinction between the Other and the self is the ultimate reduction of distinctions that defines *nihilism.* When we find people, that is, when we find ourselves totally at the disposal of the Other, and living this exposure as response to the Other by stripping the self of its egoity, like the saint, our culture tells us to label this behavior pathological, weird, freaky. But *hagiology* (the study of saints) is not the same as *teratology* (the study of freaks).

Yet we can accept this radical *alterocentrism,* this paradoxical ontological relationship between the self and the Other, where the Other is always other, the self is always the same, yet the self finds itself committed to the Other because the Other is in the self. "The soul is the Other in me" (1974/81, p. 191n3). As we overcome our cultural nihilistic bias of reducing the Other to the same of the egoic self, as we open ourselves to hagiology, we become nourished by this paradoxical inspiration.

Let me quickly try to dissuade readers from the belief that alterocentrism is a reduction of the self to an object of the Other, a slavery that encourages the Other to abuse the self. That kind of reduction of the self would *not* be a commitment to the good of the Other. Enabling the Other to violate the rights of the self would be a reduction of the Other to a monster. That would be the same nihilism as the egocentrism of our radical individualism that reduces the Other to an object to fill the needs of the self. (I will more fully try to correct this false understanding of Levinas's radical altruism later in the Interlude.)

Modern psychology as an egology has contributed to nihilistic isolation of the self from the Other. We need a psychology that would be more than an egology. We need a psukhology founded on the paradoxical relationship between the self and the separate Other where the self, remaining separate, finds itself in the Other by its commitment to the Other, remaining separate.

An Other-centered psukhology not only would go against our American cultural individualism, but, although very Jewish, very Platonic and Christian, it would also go against a philosophical tradition since the ancient Greeks, a tradition that has kept the self concentrated in its own center. Other-centeredness obviously goes against logic and reason. Especially does this alterocentrism, this radical altruism in contrast to our accustomed egocentrism, go against our natural tendency toward fulfillment of private wants. We are fearful of paradox: this paradox may call our most precious assumptions into question.

Since we know our own needs, we reduce others to that which can fill those needs. However, this radical decentering offers the foundation of a philosophy that makes possible an authentic ethics that does not reduce others. Only this *self-for-the-Other* makes sense of the experiences of the paradoxes of the weakness of power and the power of weakness. This "malady of identity," as Levinas calls it, is not only the source of our suffering, but also the source of our true identity. *Self-for-the-Other* redeems suffering.

This radical challenge to *individualism* does not, I must quickly add, support *collectivism*, as defenders of extreme individualism might fear. The self as *the-Other-in-me* challenges both the vision of the isolated individual driven by pure self-interest, as well as the notion of the person as a mere piece of a larger social structure, trapped inside determining systems. This ethical philosophy of the-Other-in-me is indeed an individualism, but a particular kind of individualism, one that attends not to the privilege of the ego, not to the rights of the ego, but to the particular and personal responsibility of the "I" for the Other. My unique individuality is not based on my particular set of qualities as properties: gender, race, ethnicity, age, religion, occupation, citizenship, political affiliation, sexual orientation, personality profile, refined skills, beauty, intelligence, honors, birth order, fingerprints, DNA coding, even my developed virtues of service, and so forth. Nor is my individuality based on my *individual rights*. It is based on my *individual responsibility*. I am I because I cannot pass off my responsibilities to any other. I cannot turn away. I cannot get outside myself being looked at by the needy Other. I am assigned responsibility, independent of my choosing.

Let me repeat the Dostoevski quote Levinas uses to express this particular individualism of responsibility and guilt: "We are all guilty of all and for all men before all, and I more than the others" (Levinas, 1982/1985, p. 98). This ethical philosophy challenges the individualism that emphasizes my individual *rights* over my individual *responsibilities*.

To say that the self is *the-Other-in-me,* or that *the center of the self is in the Other* is neither to abandon the self as lost in the collective, nor to let it be swallowed up in an exclusive union with a single other person. Neither the self nor the Other have lost their individuality, nor is either isolated from each other.

An understanding of the decentered *psukhe,* the self replaced from the center of the self, requires a more radical revolution than that called for by the astronomer at the dawn of modernity, to replace the earth as the center of the universe. Like Copernicus, who did not offer us simply a humbling theory, Levinas offers a description of ethical reality that is not a prescription to abandon autonomous selfhood, but to describe selfhood based on its responsibility to others. Although Other-centered ethics has a deep historical vein in our religious and philosophical tradition, to our modern eyes and ears, this description of the relationship between the self and the Other seems initially too extreme, too extravagant. Yet it tends to evoke in us a sense of relief, a confidence in an ethical philosophy that speaks to our experience.

De-centering is at the basis of the most fundamental paradox of the human: *The self finds its meaning, not centered in itself as an ego establishing its individual freedom and power, but as a self facing the other person who calls the self out of its center to be ethically responsible.* The freedom and power of the self is invested in the self by and for the needs of the Other. The identity of the self lies in listening to the call of others, in being touched by their absolute dignity and their vulnerability, and in using its invested freedom to respond responsibly to those others. We shall see that this fundamental enigma of the *self-from-and-for-the-Other* is at the heart of the paradox of the weakness of power and the power of weakness.

In this chapter, I focus on a few philosophical concepts of Emmanuel Levinas that provide the foundation for the contrast between *egocentrism* and *radical altruism,* what he calls *heteronomy,* between an *egology* and a *psukhology.* His philosophical works are difficult to read, yet they also evoke simple concepts. He is simultaneously complex and yet redundant when unpacking these few simple ideas. He is in dialogue with and builds upon so many philosophers that preceded him, and yet challenges nearly all of them. He clearly uses the methodology of the phenomenologists, and yet attends to the human Other that cannot be understood as a *phenomenon,* as Husserl uses the term. The Other escapes the understanding of the psyche.

I will try to be faithful to Levinas's insights about the mystery and ubiquity of the human Other to the self, and yet try to make these insights clearly understood. Because his revolutionary vision challenges the main tenets of our cultural and philosophical tradition of individualism, I present his approach in sets of distinctions, not as contradictions, but certainly as oppositions. The first side of each distinction is not criticized as wrong, only as insufficiently half the story. The second side calls the first side into question, enriches the first side by calling it into question and thus into its authentic freedom. The second side, ontologically weaker than the first, claims an ethical priority over the first.

SIX FUNDAMENTAL DISTINCTIONS

Let me first name the distinctions, and then describe Levinas's explanations.[1]

1. The experience of totality and the experience of infinity
2. Need and desire
3. Willful activity and radical passivity
4. Freedom as self-generated and self-directed and freedom as responsibility invested in the self by and for the other
5. Social equality and ethical inequality
6. The said and saying

Totality and Infinity

After the first day of volunteering at a day shelter for homeless, jobless, often crazy street people, a student wrote in her journal:

> When I walked in, I was hit with a bad odor. I looked around and everyone seemed the same. They were shabby and mostly alone. Many were asleep hunched over on chairs or curled up on pads on the floor. At first, they were all the same: they were poor; they were simply poor. . . . After a while I got to talking to a man near the coffee counter. He told me about his tough luck as a family man. . . . Another man joined us and told me he hadn't seen his daughter in twelve years. . . . After a while, they weren't all the same. I went in there expecting and seeing stereotypes. I met guys who blew my stereotypes apart. Each one had a story that was both like and not like everyone else's. Each one had more to his life than being unlucky and therefore poor.

Inspired to observe experiences by way of a phenomenology articulated by Levinas, I discover in reflection two radically different concepts:

---

1. Since I am not a Levinas scholar, but a psychologist reading his work for years and wanting to make his philosophy accessible to other psychologists and lay readers, I may fall short of the standards expected of philosophical scholarship.

totality and *infinity*. The concept of *totality* comes from the experience that "something" is *nothing-more-than* whatever my categories make of it. For example, this keyboard is nothing-more-than my tool; my bus driver is nothing-more-than part of the equipment that gets me to my destination. I find others describing the same thing: the men at the shelter were, for my student, nothing-more-than-poor. The "something" perceived is just an example of a stereotype convenient for the perceiver to make sense of his or her world.

The concept of *infinity*, on the other hand, comes from the experience that someone is *always-more-than* what I know, what I judge, what I use and enjoy, for example, always-more-than equipment, always-more-than-poor. Other persons facing me are infinitely more than a member of my convenient categories.

In my ordinary activity, getting my work done and satisfying my needs, I tend to totalize that which is needed. To organize my life, I try to *comprehend* my situation with my understanding, stay in *control* of my action, and *consume* for the enjoyment of my feelings. In my *natural attitude*[2] I am the center of my world and everything else spreads out from there. The bread I eat, the roof I seek for shelter, the tool I use, the events in my plans, these are reduced to things of my useful activity. They are for me, at this time and in this situation, absorbed in the totality I produce. They are nothing-more-than what I need. In my mundane and pragmatic life, I set aside the identity of things in themselves, and assign them identities to satisfy my needs. I make them fit universal concepts for me and ignore their particularity. It's my world; I'm in charge; I'm the center; and I'm responsible only to and for myself. There is nothing unnatural about this life of totalizing; it's the natural life of an organism. Levinas says that the ego feeds off and enjoys the world. And this feeding produces in the conscious and reflective organism the idea of *totality*.

But then my beloved wife enters on the stage of my life, or one of my children, or a student, or a stranger, or even an enemy. Although, for the sake of convenience in my hurry I tend to reduce each to a usefulness for me, they resist my tendency with their inherent autonomy and call me to attend to them as independent of my use. My totalizing attitude gets tilted, disturbed, even shocked. These people, in their particularity, get *in my face* and disrupt my world. They are not objects able to be totalized for my needs. When I totalize, I do not actually reduce them; I only succeed in

---

2. The *natural attitude* is the term the phenomenologists use to describe the condition of being pressed into nature, without reflection, without any distance from what I am doing.

reducing my own understanding of them. I don't distort them; I distort myself. I deny myself, not the Other.

Moreover, by the presence of other persons, those things I have been feeding on, the bread I eat, the roof that shelters, the tool I use, are no longer nothing-more-than objects to fill the lacks in my organism and ego. They should be called gifts I have received from the sacrifices of others, and gifts I am charged to hand over to others who have needs and rights more deserving than mine. The needs of other people command me to share these objects as gifts. I can refuse that command, of course, and find ways to justify my refusals. But I know in conscience that others' needs command me just the same. I may not know the depth of the others' needs; I may not fully know why they command me; I may not know how I could possibly fill their needs. They are always-more-than what I can know. Their needs are always-more-than what I could ever find out. But others' needs command me, haunt me, even obsess me. I sometimes think that if it were not for my skill of self-distraction and reduction of the worthiness of others, I could not fill any of my own needs. But surely I do.

So, on the one hand, the things and people of the world of my separate self are totalizable, reducible to stereotypes. On the other hand, the other person overflows my experience of her or him, and produces in me the awareness of another that is not able to be reduced to a stereotype, to a general concept. Levinas calls this awareness of always-more-than the "idea of infinity." He calls the effort to fit something into my stereotype, the awareness of nothing-more-than, the "idea of totality." On the one hand, the idea of totality is produced in the experience of objects needed, grasped, passed around from hand to hand, named in language, comprehended, controlled, and consumed. On the other hand, the idea of infinity is produced in the experience of the other person as essentially *un*comprehendable, *un*controllable, and *un*consumable. The other person exceeds my grasp, cannot be reduced, cannot be totalized by a concept or label or any effort by me to use her or him. I too often try to reduce others, and I have a kind of operational success in this reduction. But I fail not because of my lack of skill or effort, but because of the Other's inherent resistance to be totalized.

The concept of totality is convenient; it serves me well in my natural and socially evolved drive for self-preservation. The concept of totality creates the possibility of all science and technology, philosophy and psychology, economics of self-interest, partisan politics, wars, compromised peace, and events of power against weakness. The concept of totality creates the possibility for all abstract theory, empirical observation, labor, manufacturing, possession of objects, commercial exchange, enjoyment of goods, sharing them, bickering over them, hoarding them, destroying them, and killing others for them. The concept of totality provides the arena for the social intercourse of daily life, especially when paradoxes turn into conflict.

It seems I live my ordinary life within the realm of totality. But I am called by infinity, the infinite worthiness and neediness of others, to be ethically responsible while I fulfill my own needs—no, even before I fill my own needs!

Although the infinity of others calls me to respond to their needs (and, certainly, everyone is needy, from the poorest to the richest), the concept of infinity is the separation of the self from the Other. The infinity of the Other puts that person beyond my grasp. The Other is truly *other*, and I am *I* (what Levinas calls the *same*). The experience of the Other as radically other, irreducibly other, is the recognition of her or his inherent dignity, the intrinsic worth of the Other, not derived from my needs or from my evaluation and judgment of the Other's qualities. The self does not decide and assign the otherness of the Other, nor does it bestow dignity on the Other by measuring her or him against some quality wished for by the self. The experience of the Other's infinity protects the Other from my need to reduce her or him. The Other is irreducible. The Other, as other, commands dignity. The Other's worthiness is not the result of my astute judgment. The Other's worthiness is absolute: ab-solved (washed from, cleansed of) my ego-centered judgments. The Other reveals her or his dignity to my immediate psychological experience. The concept of infinity is not my idea; it is a gift to me from the *always-more-than* of the Other.

The self, wrapped in its ego, without doubt, often misses this revelation. But this *epiphany* (an understanding shown to me and not produced by me) of the Other as an independent dignity is revealed to the immediate perception by the self. There is no need to argue the Other's worth by a logic founded on a premise of some *ontology of Being*, or some *theology of creatureliness*, and certainly not some *economics of comparative productivity*. The face of the Other, the very presence before my tendency to totalize, is the origin of the experience of infinity. The origin and compelling mandate of the experience of infinity does not come from my rational intellect. This concept of infinity is a pre-rational and generous gift. Infinity is revealed to be a transcendental condition for rationality.

One critic of Levinas, Jacques Derrida, argues that this claim that the Other shows herself as having infinite worth is an "empiricism" (Derrida, 1964). The philosophy of empiricism is defined as an approach that points out the presence of things without giving the necessary and sufficient reasons for their presence. Rationalist critics of empiricism say it is an intellectual scandal not to rationally prove the existence of something.[3] That neither Levinas nor anyone else has philosophically proven that our neighbor is infinitely worthy is not an intellectual scandal. The scandal is that daily we see, hear, or read about people violating the inherent dignity of others. We do not first need the rational arguments of human worth before we are shocked by events showing *homo homini lupus,* "man is a wolf to man." The demand for a philosophical proof that others have inherent dignity and that we are responsible for them is a rationalism that has brutalized millions of people.

The relationship between myself and the Other is infinitely beyond my comprehension, control, and consumption. Every relationship is, as Levinas says, a relationship like no other relationship. Others are infinitely far away from me: their otherness is absolutely other; and yet others are infinitely nearby: their neediness commands my individual responsibility without my being able ethically to escape. We are commanded, "let the Other be," and simultaneously, "serve the Other." The face of the Other, without needing to speak, says "Do not do violence to me!" and, also, "Provide for my needs!" This experience of the infinite worthiness of the Other, and of her or his commanding needs, is at the heart of a fundamental psychological paradox: the Other is always beyond me, and always calling me.

Furthermore, the Other's call is addressed to an infinite responsibility: the more I provide, the more I am called. Levinas says, "the better I accomplish my duty, the fewer rights I have; the more I am just, the more guilty I am" (1961/1969, p. 244). At the heart of this psukhological experience lies not only the recognition of paradox, but also the suffering of paradox. The *Other-in-me* is my *malady of identity.* Suffering is at the heart of the paradox of the power of weakness. But this relationship of an infinite responsibility that is always-more-than what I can ever accomplish is a sublime suffering; it is love.

Kierkegaard described the *angst* of human existence as the tenuousness of Being itself. Nonbeing, death will find and surprise each of us. Levinas points out another threat to absolute contentment: the death of others, my complicity, my inability to save them or to even keep them from dying alone, my inability to know if my understanding of others and my generous efforts do anything more than make me feel good about those efforts. The angst of human existence rests in a kind of deep-seated

---

3. I am not defending classical empiricism, the claim that reason can be reduced to sense data. Maurice Merleau-Ponty's astute criticism of both empiricism and rationalism in his *Phenomenology of Perception,* 1962, is the argument I follow.

skepticism: I never know the value of my behavior for others. This constitutes my existential anxiety: I know I am responsible, and yet I am uncertain of my responses. I know I am called to generous service. This call
pulls me both to the sublimity and to the suffering of responsibility. Just
as the satisfied person is not one who has no needs, but rather one who
has fulfilled needs, yet only temporarily fulfilled; so the happy person is
not one who is not called or hears no call, but the one who responds as
well as possible, yet suffers the *insomnia* of "never enough." As
Kierkegaard uses the word "angst" to define human existence, so Levinas
uses the word "insomnia" to define the uncertainty of completion of
responsibility. I can never rest assured.

Let me reintroduce my concern about our science of psychology.
Psychology seems to focus on the ego fulfilling its needs. From this perspective, everything else can be described as potentially either fulfilling
those needs or making those needs stronger. Modern psychology tends to
be reductionistic. It reduces the self to a complex of hungers or drives.
Psychology reduces the experience of others to an event of the ego knowing or feeling about others as objects that can or cannot fulfill the needs of
the ego. Psychology thus reduces the primary experience of the absolute
infinity of the Other to a *totalizable* event of nature. It is too often an objec-
tivistically inspired science of generalizations, a set of labels placed on
processes and states, on properties of human behavior. To the extent that
psychology fails to remain faithful to the experience of the distinction
between totality and infinity, then it remains an egology, the study of an
isolated ego totalizing everything other than itself, confined within the
contentment of its own making, and thereby condemned to self-sabotage.

The distinction of Levinas between totality and infinity provides the
foundation for a nonegological psukhology, where the psukhe, breath,
soul of life, is inspired by the dignity and needs of others into the paradoxical self: inspired but unsure of itself. This psukhology could study the
styles of the individual assignments and responses, the styles of listening
to the call and responsibly responding, as well as the styles of "turning
away from" and abusing the call of the Other. Psychology ought to return
to being a moral science and practice.

Need and Desire

In one of those encounter groups where I found myself during the early
seventies, a wife finally shouted back to her wimpy husband,

> Whenever you insist that you *need* me, I feel like one of your nec-
> essary tools or toys, like your car, or your golf clubs, or that
> damn overstuffed chair you've claimed. You make me feel like
> you do not want me because of me, but you need me for you.

Her complaint is not uncommon. When we say we *need* our loved ones, we think we are expressing as strongly as possible how much we love them. But the more emphasis we put on our expression of *need*—the longer the list of indispensable qualities and behavior of the beloved—the more the Other feels used, the greater the burden the Other feels. Certainly we have needs that the partner helps fill. But the beloved is loved, desired for her own sake, not just as a provider for the ego's needs.

The distinction between *need* and *desire*, articulated by Levinas (1961/1969), helps us understand this paradox of power and weakness. Egological psychology, having missed the distinction between *totality* and *infinity*, reducing the Other person to the totalizing category of an object of need, cannot distinguish between *need* and *desire*.

A need is directed toward things. What is needed is what is lacking. The needed object is totalized to that thing which can fill the lack. Needs urge me to make what is not me into me. To fill a need, at the cognitive level I understand (sometimes misunderstand) a thing to fit my need; at the behavioral level, I take it and move (sometimes fumble) it to fill my need; at the affective level, I receive from the thing the satisfaction (sometimes dissatisfaction) I needed. Even with other persons my needs urge me to *comprehend* (reduce others to my cognitive grasp of things), *control* (make others fit my particular behavioral project), and *consume* (find in others a goodness, not for their sake, but for what I can sustain myself and affectively enjoy).

Desire is different from need. Desire is directed to the good of other persons. Desire is love.[4] The desired does not fill a need, but rather deepens desire. Desire for the Other, the independent other, cannot be satisfied; desire enriches me in its unquenchable concerns and caresses. Desire does not wish to comprehend, control, and consume, to take the Other into the self, but to be with the Other as the Other exists as an wholly separate person. Desire does not wish to make the Other fit the needs of the self, but reaches out to the Other to provide for the Other's needs as those needs are expressed to the self.

When I find myself using the Other, stereotyping her or him, manipulating her or him, expecting too much of her or him, and sometimes getting satiated and bored with her or him, I must admit I have turned my relationship of desire into an ego-centered need. My needs want the Other

---

4. For now, we can use the word *love* as an equivalent of *desire*. However, Levinas made a distinction between *desire* and *love*. Love seeks the relationship with the beloved excluding others so the Other can attend to the self. Desire, on the other hand, does not exclude other Others. They are implied in the desire for the Other. Desire seeks the good of the Other without any interest in fulfilling some need of the self by the desired one, and therefore seeks the good for all others.

to be my thing-like image, rather than as the absolutely Other who she or he is.

Descriptions of personal altruistic experiences so frequently contain statements like, "I feel I got more out of helping others than what I could give to them." This is a legitimate admission, but it does not make altruistic experiences reducible to occasions of need-fulfillment. To claim that the altruistic event of serving only fulfills ego-needs reduces our most sublimely experienced motive: *desire*. We can distinguish between need and desire by recognizing that the origin of desire arises from the independent goodness of the desired, while the origin of need grows out of the lack of some good within the self. It is precisely because the origin of desire comes from the Other that we experience its sublimity over the fulfillment of needs, whose origins come from the self. The desire for the Other calls us to transcend our own needs, to go beyond our organismic and egological self.

We often use these terms (need and desire) the other way around: we say we need other people; and we desire things. This may be a semantic problem: we often use the word *desire* to mean either a very strong need or a sexual drive. More likely, this reversal of meanings shows that none of our desires are pure. Even when we most righteously try to respect the dignity of the Other, we mix in a bit of totalizing to fill a selfish need. We still have needs and we lapse into using the other person as a needed object, not respecting them as worthy and independent of our needs.

Or we might argue that reversing the terms demonstrates a social pathology. In our affluent culture of "cancerous individualism," described so well by Bellah and his colleagues (*Habits of the Heart*, 1986), we are taught, on the one hand, to reduce other people to objects needed: we act as if we could consume them. We are taught by our culture, on the other hand, to desire material things: we become pathologically driven to things. We insatiably consume and idolatrously honor possessions.

When the human sciences theoretically reduce the experience of *desire* to the notion of *need*, as does much of psychology, sociology, economics, and political science (everything is explainable by them in terms of self-interest), they do so by a nihilistic reduction of the distinction between totality and infinity. These sciences must recognize that needs seek objects able to be totalized in a definition of utility that reduces them to what fills a lack. Distinct from need, desire seeks that which is always infinitely beyond us, absolutely non-totalizable. While need unites things with the ego, desire discovers the other person infinitely far away and paradoxically infinitely close to the self, closer to the self than the self.

Willful Activity and Radical Passivity

Accuse someone of being *passive* and you will likely get hit with an highly *active* response. The very word *passive* has come to describe an indignity, insulting to people in our self-empowered, aggressive society. The adjective *active*, on the other hand, is flattering. *Active* is a power word. It sells. It is used in advertising as much as "new and improved." *Passive* is weak, denied, disgusting to active people. A friend once told me how much he hates the word *passive* and any word associated with it. He even bristles at road signs that say, YIELD. In this cultural condition we must examine the paradoxical notion of *passivity*.

Levinas describes our reception of the command of the Other to be responsible as "a passivity—but it is a passivity beneath all passivity" (1969, p. 101). This command, passively experienced by me, not chosen by me, makes my authentic activity a *radical passivity*, and my passivity an activity: I am called without choice (passive) to serve (active) the needs of the other. When I turn away (active) from the Other, I retreat into self-obsession, self-compulsion, self-indulgence (passive).

This third distinction of Levinas disturbs the egology of traditional philosophy and psychology, as well as our popular culture of individual competition. To be more philosophically specific, Levinas distinguishes *intentionality of consciousness* (activity) from the *nonintentionality of affectivity*:[5] enjoyment, suffering, and the for-the-other of conscience (passivity).

The father of phenomenology, Edmund Husserl, described the human as "consciousness constituting its world." He used the term "intentionality" to indicate how human consciousness actively *intends out* toward the world and makes the things in the world meaningful for consciousness. The metaphor of the flashlight has been helpful to clarify the intentionality of consciousness. When I direct the light beam on the bike in my dark basement, I do not make it pop into existence. The bike was there in the dark before the flashlight and I came down the stair. We, the bicycle and I with flashlight, only *disclose* the bike already there. Intentionality, like the light beam, is the way consciousness (that which knows) discloses the objects of consciousness (that which is known). Consciousness as intentional is a form of the voluntary: it is a chosen activity of the ego. The phenomenologists challenge the exaggerated egoism and activity claimed by

---

5. See Andrew Tallon's "Nonintentional Affectivity, Affective Intentionality, and the Ethical in Levinas's Philosophy," in *Ethics as First Philosophy: The Significance of Emmanuel Levinas for Philosophy, Literature, and Religion* (1995, pp. 107–21).

philosophical Idealism. Idealism is that school of philosophy that reduces the objects of knowing to nothing more than the pure product of the consciousness of the ego. For the Idealists, the flashlight beam (consciousness) would make the bicycle come into existence. The phenomenology of Husserl, on the other hand, describes knowing as "co-constitution" between the world of things and consciousness. The thing and I cooperate in forming the *meaning* I have of the thing.

Levinas thinks the description of consciousness offered by Husserl puts too much emphasis on the activity of the consciousness of the ego, particularly in knowing the Other. He thinks Husserl is too influenced by the Western tradition of egology, too influenced by Idealism. Levinas would generally agree with Husserl's phenomenological description of human knowing. He philosophically disagrees with Husserl's and with other phenomenologists' implication that intentional (active) consciousness is the only relationship the self has with that which is other than the self, especially other humans. Phenomenologists do not recognize a nonintentional (radically passive) relationship with other persons.[6]

Conscience, the call to seek good and avoid evil, is, for the phenomenologists, a kind of active intentional consciousness of the ego. Having my ethical obligation disclosed by me is a form of my active knowing, rather than a form of my being passively commanded by the Other, as it is for Levinas. For Husserl, I disclose my duty to myself. I decide my obligations. For Levinas, my duty is revealed to me. If I hold the notion that my obligation to feed my children was arrived at solely by my generous will, insisting it was not an obligation passively assigned me by their hunger, Levinas would consider me arrogantly self-deceived. Yet our individualism wants to insist on an ideological conviction that we are the origin of our assignments.

For Levinas, conscience is much more passive than ethicists describe. This passivity of conscience is not like Freud's superego in which the forming of conscience is the automatic interiorization or introjection of the parents' and culture's values, demands, and prohibitions. Levinas's notion of the passivity of conscience is founded on the experience that the face of the Other calls my egoism into question. The Other challenges my effort to comprehend (stereotype her), my effort to control (use her for my plans), and my effort to consume (enjoy her as a thing). The Other tells me, simply by her presence, that these are violations of her radical Otherness, of her infinite dignity, of her worthiness independent of my judgments and decisions. The source of the challenge to my tendency toward vio-

---

6. I think Merleau-Ponty was on the way to the notion of *passivity*, but he died before he could describe it as Levinas does.

lence is not my "intentional constituting consciousness," my mental activity, deciding to question my own tendencies. I cannot police myself. The source of my conscience is the Other's goodness challenging me as usurping her rights by misunderstanding her, by using her, and by enjoying goods that she needs more than I. I do not *construct* my conscience. I do not *do it*; it *happens* to me! I do not so much *actively* form my conscience on my own, as it is *passively* formed. My conscience is passively formed by the independent goodness of the Other instructing me about her goodness, and commanding me to be responsible. I do not choose my fundamental responsibility. It is assigned to me simply by being a neighbor to my neighbor, by being a being that is vulnerable to being called, by being human.

Of course, with my free will, I may choose to accept or not accept the individual responsibility assigned to me, or rather choose to accept my responsibility by not being generous. I know I have the freedom, the possibility, the license to choose to accept or not. I have past experiences in my life in which I have chosen to act irresponsibly by forgetting, turning away, neglecting, even abusing others. I also have experiences in which I acted responsibly by remembering, turning toward, serving, and even sacrificing myself for the Other. My response is not determined like a force in nature. I am *commanded* to be responsible precisely because I am not *caused* to be responsible. My conscience is neither the superego deposited in me by parents and causing me to do certain actions, nor the noble psychological structure of good intentions on which I too often falsely pride myself. Conscience is initially passively received. The psyche is still the psyche, the free agent, but this freedom is commanded independent of its self-initiated and self-directed freedom. It is commanded by the Other. The psyche in the soul is the Other in me.

Levinas indicates that the origin of nonintentional conscience can be traced to the experience of a nonintentional affectivity of sensible enjoyment. Enjoyment should not be considered a kind of active intentional consciousness. Enjoyment is certainly passive, for instance, when I eat ice cream, I don't decide to enjoy it. I enjoy it as a gift. Enjoyment is unexpected and undeserved, certainly not constituted by an ego. The actual enjoyment of anything pleasing is always better, or worse, than the anticipation, the expectation in the consciousness of the ego. As the menu cannot be equivalent to the meal, so the memory of the past enjoyment cannot be equivalent to the enjoyment in the act of eating. The actual enjoyment always surprises, always overflows my constituted knowledge, my image of its possible enjoyment. Even when I don't enjoy what I anticipated I would enjoy, this surprise is an overflowing, a passive reception.

Enjoyment overflows the ego, graces our eating, our looking, hearing, all our affectivity.

Furthermore, enjoyment is undeserved. It is not a payment for my good work. I may deserve payment or favor for work under some economic or social agreement, but the enjoyment of the reward is an independent gift. It is gratuitous. I am passive to enjoyment. Thank God! This may be difficult for us to accept in this age of our obsession with the idea of "deservedness." But we sabotage enjoyment by claiming it is deserved. Enjoying the pure gift of the good, surprising and unmerited, makes up the joy of life.

However, the very possibility of passive enjoyment points to the human vulnerability of being denied satisfaction: suffering. Suffering is certainly passive. It is gratuitous. Suffering is unexpected and undeserved, certainly not chosen by my intentional consciousness. We are vulnerable, exposed to otherness, otherness that can hurt as well as give enjoyment. When we suffer for nothing, we recognize that the passivity of the sensible cannot be turned into activity.

Finally, this very enjoyment and suffering, this passive exposedness to the Other, is the basis of our *conscience*. Although enjoyment allows for the ego to be complacent in itself, to be exempt from interpersonal tensions, to experience the privateness of the ego, at least for a while, the experiences of enjoyment and suffering provide the conditions for the *self-for-the-Other*. Conscience, the calling to responsibility for the needs of the Other, is founded on sensibility, not on some rational category of constituting consciousness. In empathy, I do not go through some syllogistic reasoning such as:

When I need things, I suffer.
Since he is just like me, *another me*, he needs things.
Since he is just like me, *another me*, he must be suffering.
I should share my things.

The immediacy and passivity of the sensible is the immediacy and passivity of enjoyment and suffering, and is the immediacy and passivity of feeling the suffering of the Other, and the desire to give. While the Other is *not another me*, the Other is proximate to me, closer to me than I am to me; the Other is in me. The Other's proximity (the Other in the self) calls me to empathy, calls me to give of my material self. Giving "is not a gift of the heart (reason), but of the bread from one's mouth" (Levinas, 1981, p. 74).

The origin of moral conscience is in the passivity of sensibility, as Levinas would have it, rather than in the activity of reason, as Kant would have it. To help us understand this description, let me turn to Maurice Merleau-Ponty's description of perception or sensibility (1964, pp.

96–155). He shows how the happiness or sadness or anger of the other person is perceived or sensed, rather than reasoned about. When I see the turned-up corners of her mouth and her widened eyes, I know that she is happy. How do I know she is experiencing happiness? My ego tells me to use the following sequences of reason:

When my mouth corners turn up and my eyes widen, I am happy.

I can solve the equation: Since she is *another me*, my bodily appearance is to my experience of happiness, as her bodily appearance is to her experience.

Therefore, when I see her body appear like this, I reason that she is experiencing happiness just like me.

This seems reasonable. But Merleau-Ponty points out two flaws in this reasoning (1964, pp. 113–120). It is both (*a*) contrary to experience, and (*b*) self-contradictory.

(*a*) I do not experience going through this first syllogistic premise: my body is to my experience as her body is to her experience; and follow the second premise: I can compare my body with her body; and then conclude: therefore when I see her look like me, then I reason that she experiences as I do. Psychologists, defending their egology, would say that, although we do not clearly experience this process of reason because we do it too quickly, and on the unconscious level, our psyche does this reasoning. But their reasoning is still unfounded on experience. I do not have an image of what I look like when I smile from happiness to compare to my perception of the Other's smile, to reason that she is happy. Frankly I do not know what I look like when I am happy. Even when I try to mimic in the mirror, it is a fake smile. I am unaware of the appearance of my smiling face. Although I feel my face move when I smile, this feeling of muscles and skin cannot be used as the equivalent of the appearance of the smile of the other. I see her happiness expressed in her smile. I do not see skin shape by muscle movement. Her smile is her happiness. The old body-mind split of the egological rationalists is not experienced in my life with my neighbor.

(*b*) The line of reasoning from self-experience to Other-experience is also contradictory. I have to know the Other's appearance of happiness in order to match it with my experience of my own happiness. I have to use as my first premise (my perception of her happiness) what I am trying to conclude (her happiness). Not fair logic! I do not see signs of happiness and conclude they are signs of happiness. I see *meanings* expressed by others, in this example, her happiness. This is the insight given us by the phenomenologists: Husserl, Merleau-Ponty, and others: *perception* grasps *meanings*. Perception is not the tool of reason. Psychology's prejudice toward reducing perception to an act of "quick, unconscious, and previously learned reason" is the product of an egology. Reason is the dominating tool of the ego. But perception is the way we, who are vulnerable, passively receive the meanings of the world. We do not want to admit that we are passive. We want active control, especially rationally active control. So under the influence of an egological prejudice, we describe perception as a poor descendant of reason. Recovering an understanding of the primacy of perception (using the great insights of Husserl, Merleau-Ponty, and others), the primacy of sensibility would be an essential project of psukhology.

A developmental psychology founded on an egology would say that as an adult I have learned from past experiences the signs of others' happiness. But if I cannot appeal to my own appearance in present time; even less can I appeal to past experiences of reading happiness on the face of previous others. I would have to push these experiences back to even prior experiences, finally to my infancy, when I recognized the happiness of my mother. This is where Merleau-Ponty offers us very helpful insights. Certainly the infant who smiles back at its mother's smile does not go through the syllogism: "My bodily appearance is to my experience of happiness, as mother's bodily appearance is to mother's experience of happiness. Therefore, when I see mom's body appear like this, show these signs, I reason that she is happy." The infant does not reason like this. All perception, for the infant and the adult is of *meaning*, not *signs* pointing to meaning constructed by reason out of the blocks of percepts.

We perceive the happiness, sadness, anger, and so forth of others. We often make mistakes, but these mistakes only show that these emotional meanings are perceived rather than reasoned. Likewise, I perceive through sensibility the suffering of the Other, and perceive that suffering as a call to me to be responsible. The reasoning of Kant, "This person before me is a human; humans should not be used as means, but only as ends in themselves; therefore I should not use this person, but should treat her or him as having dignity of her or his own accord," is self-contradictory. How do I know that this object before me is a person? Not because he has a similar appearance to the me whom I primarily know to be a person. Maybe he is a manikin with an appearance of a person but not a person. Rather I know him as a person because I perceive his worthiness independent of my judgments of him. I see, hear, even touch, smell, and taste him enjoying life, being angry, sad, or frustrated, being a free, independent existence filled with his own life. I do not, with my reason, judge him to be a free and happy or sad person; I perceive him this way. Merleau-Ponty's description of the primacy of perception over reason powerfully elucidates Levinas's description of the primacy of passive perception over active reason in understanding the dignity and call of the Other.

Levinas offers extraordinary descriptions of enjoyment. His philosophy of responsibility, even sacrifice for others, cannot be called an asceticism. As I immediately experience the good of enjoyment, without a detour through my rationalizing consciousness, I similarly experience the accusation by the Other's needs against my egocentrism, and my responsibility to give her the bread from my mouth. The ethical call is therefore not from a rational conclusion, a Kantian categorical imperative. Ethics originates in nonintentional sensibility: my enjoyment, her need, her nonintentional accusation and inspiration to me, my hearing her call, all are passively given before my reason must figure out how to respond.

This passivity of affectivity is not the equivalent of mechanical passivity, where an effect is the passive result of the cause. Affective passivity is more passive than mechanical passivity because it is the passivity of meaning. I receive a meaning, a nonintentional, gratuitous meaning that delights me or pains me. I receive the call to responsibility from and for the Other. This *radical passivity* to the *radical otherness of the Other* is the origin of my conscience.

Emphasis on the passivity of conscience over the activity of consciousness and conscience, and the emphasis of enjoyment/suffering of the psyche over the power/weakness of the ego is important in defining a psukhology that is not a narrow egology. To supremely recognize our vulnerability to the Other person would help us to understand not only the suffering we inflict on each other, but also the gifts we give each other. We need a psukhology of gratitude, the study of the soul experiencing the Other *breathed into* the self. We need a psukhology of our radical social connectedness and identity, to balance our understanding of our isolated identity, a psukhology of commitment to balance our individualism, a psukhology of responsibility to balance our competitiveness.

Self-Initiated Freedom and Invested Freedom

Personal freedom has been placed at the top of the hierarchy of values in most theoretical systems that explain the psychological, sociological, economic, and political life of humans, certainly Western humans. These hierarchies map the energy of the life of the self separated from others. Enjoying pleasure in the midst of its acquired goods, the self is at home with itself honoring its personal freedom. The life of the separated individual is found in enjoyment of goods. Needs are not a burden to the self. Fulfilled needs are the enjoyment of life. No doubt about it, because of our needs, we find ourselves dependent upon material things. But it is a happy dependence. I'm pleased that my digestive system transforms into nutrients and wastes the contents of my recent meal. I love the taste of groceries. To continually consume needed things brings happiness; happiness supports our freedom.

But the bliss of feeding off the world is not the end. First of all, the bliss is ephemeral, short-lived and often traitorous, as when my diet is bad. Secondly, the self privately filling its needs and enjoying life recognizes that other people provide this life of enjoyment. The self is not self-sufficient, not that separated from others. The world of material things needed and enjoyed by the self are gifts from others given to the self and often sacrificed out of those others' own needs and desire. Not only are goods given as gifts, not only are talents and opportunities given as gifts, but, most important, others give me my very own freedom to be used responsibly to serve others. Freedom in the form of open possibilities, usable goods, developed talents, even desires, are invested in me by others. Additionally, the investment of freedom in me by others obliges me to use this freedom to serve them in their need. Responsibility, the duty to give of my understanding, my effort, and even the bread from my mouth is the fundamental call to authenticity.

Let me anticipate objections to this radical notion of *invested freedom* from the ethical philosophy of Levinas. Let me say what this paradigm shift from an egology to a radical alterology, this revolutionary turn from an ego-centered psychology to an Other-centered psukhology is not. (I will later discuss the limits to altruism more fully in the Interlude.)

First, a shift from an egology to the study of an Other-centered self is not a moral command coming from me, or from Levinas, or from some church, governing body, or familial, tribal, or other social institution. The philosophy of Levinas is not a heteronomy where I am the slave to tyrannical masters. It is not a moral system he has devised. Rather it is a description of human existence. It is a phenomenology that describes what we all see and expect others to see, and that causes us to worry about those who say they don't see. What we see is undeniable responsibility, not to the power of a social institution, but to the neediness of the face of the Other. The claim of Levinas that ethics takes priority over an ego-centered ontology is not a moralistic prescription; it is a description. Or better, it is a prescription, but a prescription revealed by the face of needy others facing me, articulated in our description of our desire for the infinite goodness of others. Levinas offers not some popular brand of theocentrism handed down from a religious hierarchy, or a presumptuous *moral majority*. Rather he describes an anthropocentrism. Not an egocentric anthropocentrism; but an altero-centric anthropo-centrism. His anthropocentrism is *re-ligious* in that notion of *re-binding* to an Absolute Other by way of rebinding to others. God is found in our committed service to others, not through a vertical and insulated conduit stretching up to a distant Transcendence.

Second, this call for a shift from an egoism to an alterocentric ethics is not a call to an asceticism that accuses us of sin in fulfilling our needs, and demands pain to make up in reparation for past or future evil pleasure. Recognizing the priority of the desire for the Other over my need for things does not make needs the root of evil. The self finds happiness filling its needs—and then finds itself called out of its enjoyment by the needs of the Other. This desire for the Other arises not from a self pulling itself out of the midst of its enjoyable needs, to an ascetic self in the midst of its ascetic needs. Desire for the Other wants the good for the sake of the Other.

Third, this desire for the goodness of the Other is not a self-righteous altruism. Altruism too often bespeaks the beliefs and practices of do-gooders who decide what the good for others ought to be, and intrude on those others to bring this good to them. Because self-righteous, pushy do-gooders have so tainted the essentially good word *altruism*, we often avoid that word, losing its proper use: a habitual style of disinterested generosity.

Two comments about altruism. First, the do-gooder is often fulfilling his own needs. He is going out to the other person for the sake of his own ego, rather than to the neediness and worthiness of the Other. This do-gooder uses the other person's neediness, consumes the other person's neediness, fulfills the needs of his self with the neediness of the Other. The Other-centered altruist is interested in the good of the Other for the sake of the Other, not for himself.

Secondly, ego-centered altruistic persons believe themselves to have within themselves the power to fulfill the needs of the Other. This implies that they know just what the Other's needs are, that they comprehend the Other, are able to place the Other's needs into a neat and previously known category. But the Other-centered altruist knows the Other is beyond his knowing. When we allow the Other to reveal who she is, we experience her as always-more-than what the self can know. We desire the Other, we are called out of ourselves to serve the needs of the Other, but we never know whether we have adequately served or could ever adequately serve her needs. Deep within our relationship to the Other lies a self-skepticism. We never totally know! The Other's needs and pleasures and requests for service are always beyond our totalizing comprehension. The paradoxical proximity and distance of the Other catches us in a conflict and humbles us.

Finally, this giving priority to the Other over the egocentric self does not mean allowing ourselves to be abused by the Other. We do not serve the Other by supporting their tendency toward abusiveness. To be ethically responsible is not, in today's language, to be codependently supporting the Other's self- and Other-destructive habits. Giving priority to others is not permitting them to abuse me or others, not my child, wife, stranger, even my enemy. On the contrary, disallowing another's abusive behavior serves not only the possible victims, but also the potential abuser.[7]

Where Levinas articulates the philosophical vision of the Other centered in the self, he claims to find the most humane aspect of the life of the human. He, and other religious geniuses, wise women and men, secular and religious saints, inspire us to listen to the call to ethical responsibility spoken to us by the neediness and worthiness of others. They call us to our incarnational authenticity. Responsibility is in our nature, hidden at times by our false obsessions with power. Robert Bellah and associates found in their research, described in *Habits of the Heart* (1985), a second language of altruism crowded out by our first language of individualism. Their subtitle, *Individualism and Commitment in Americal Life*, points to their discovery that American individualism can potentially eat us up from the inside, like immature, rapidly growing cancerous cells. On the other hand, they often found that American individualism has another side to it. We do commit ourselves to others. We are a society of joiners, of volunteers, of charitable givers, devoted to families, neighbors, churches, clubs. Tremendous generosity lies in the human heart, an openness to extraordinary sacrifice for the well-being of others, an ethical center in the lives of nearly all of us.

Psychology, wandering away from the original meaning of the psukhe in *psukhology*, has defaulted into an *egology*. Psychology needs to scratch beneath the surface of its self-need-centered theories to find the *desire* within all of us to serve the *needs* of others. Psychologists, trying to be objective scientists, have been telling themselves over and over that they must be a-valuative. They have complied so much with the dictate of science to be morally neutral that they have been reluctant to recognize the psychological experiences of the human psyche called to responsibility. Psychologists have too forcefully told themselves that descriptions of responsibility should be left to the philosopher, the theologian, and the saints, while they stay clear of any descriptions of ethical experience,

---

7. In the Interlude I will discuss the limitations placed on the self in its efforts to be ethical in the social situations where other Others are involved.

which, they warn, would inevitably turn into moralism and would taint the science.

Without moralizing, the phenomenological descriptions of Levinas tell us we have not only permission, but an obligation, according to our fundamental ethical nature, to describe moral experiences. Saints, the countless generous people we find working away to serve the needs of others without moralizing, inspire us to ethical responsibility.

Social Equality and Ethical Inequality

A basic and prized value of our modern democratic and individualistic society is *equality*. Within this culture, I cannot place myself above any other, and no one can place herself above me. Yet we all have a more primary experience, a humble honesty not to place oneself and the Other on an equal plane. The difference of the Other—not that difference defined by gender, age, race, ethnicity, religion—but that difference as individually and infinitely Other, is *absolute*. We are infinitely unequal. The Other is always infinitely more than "just another me."

Certainly, the Other cannot place herself above me by claims of talent or birthright or any other quality. Still, I must place her above me by the claim on my ethical responsibility. To claim I cannot recognize the rights of the Other over me, is to be ego-centered. In full and honest humility, the Other comes first. Levinas points out the immediate experience, "what I permit myself to demand of myself is not comparable with what I have the right to demand of the Other" (1969, p. 53). While the Other should not abuse me, this claim is not because I have rights over or equal to the other. I cannot reduce the Other to my level. Others present themselves as always more than I can know, especially more than what I know by my limited understanding of my own limited self. I have *political equality* with others, founded on a constitution and laws, but I do not have *ethical equality*, founded on the experience of rights and responsibilities in the face-to-face meeting. "Others come before me." We've heard this statement from saints and other ethical geniuses. It is a hard saying. But it is a truth that Levinas describes. It is not a truth I can insist others follow. The "Others come before me" is a truth for the me.

The Said and Saying

This fundamental inequality is expressed by Levinas when he distinguishes between what he calls the *said*, and what he calls *saying*. The *said* is the language of equality, our talk within a system of words representing concepts to which we have become accustomed in society. In much of my ordinary talk, I repeat those ideas that I have heard and read. The *said* is used to put myself forth out of my *conatus essendi*, my "will to be." When I speak the language of the *said*, I am using the commonly understood notions of an individual establishing an identity in a society of others establishing their identity. The structures of institutional society are founded on the network of the language of the *said*. It is the language of the established, and I use it to establish my place among the established. I speak of my accomplishments, my ambitions, my judgments of others, my values. I assume my listener shares these notions of how individuals establish identities. These are from the language of power in a system that is founded on an equality of opportunity.

Saying, on the other hand, is a more original communication than the *said*; we might even say it is pre-original. *Saying* is my expression inspired by the proximity (always commanding presence) and distance (always beyond my comprehension, control, and consuming) of the Other. *Saying* does not originally come from me as a freely initiated activity. It comes from me as a prevoluntary response to the Other's calling me to responsibility. I cannot first say what my responsibility is. My responsibility is commanded of me before I establish my social territory, including what I think are my regions of responsibility. *Saying* is my expression communicated to the Other's questioning my statements of the *said*, my excuses justified by an ideology that claims I am equal to the Other.

I am called to *say*. But my *saying* is my response simply by being present to the Other. I am not present the way a stick or stone is *there*. I am a human who is *there*, present to the Other, the one whose psukhe has been breathed into me by others for the sake of others. My *thereness* is not reducible to the *being there* concerned with itself, as Heidegger says in *Being and Time*. My *thereness* is the *being there* answerable to the Other. The neediness of the Other cannot turn to the stick or stone and expect responsibility. The neediness of the Other can turn to me and expect me to help, without having to ask whether I am more than a stick. The expression of the Other is the humanness of the Other calling me to *say* back to the Other "Here I am," before I calculate and claim my equal rights, even before I can form the words with my mouth "Here I am." I hear the Other revealing to me, "Here I am, worthy of dignity independent of your judgments of equality." The mouth of the Other and my ears need not be involved. The presence of the Other is the original *saying*.

When the other confronts me, faces me with neediness, challenges my claim to my rights over my responsibilities, reveals to me an obligation that is older than any promise or denial I made in earlier statements, when the face of the Other faces me, then I recognize that my *saying* "Here I am" is more original than any other originality I can speak. *Saying* is not rooted in ordinary time. It is *saying* not in the present as a remembrance of the past, nor is it an anticipation of the future. The revelation to me of the neediness of the Other is *always immediate*, and therefore timeless, *always concrete*, and therefore never deniable. It is more undeniable than the impediment that blocks my way. My saying "Here I am" is the expression to the Other that I have undeniably witnessed their presence before me. I cannot shirk the responsibility of the claim of the Other on me. I am more passive to the revelation of the Other than any passivity of receiving a blow on my head, or a subpoena from court. This revelation is not directed to me as a general member of a species, tribe, family, or citizen obligated by law in a system of equal members. It is not directed to me as one who has the ability and time from an occupational role to provide serviceable action. This revelation is addressed to me as the individual who is assigned fundamental responsibility prior to any claim to be capable and moral. It is assigned because I am the one *there*. My *thereness* is established by the face of the Other facing me, appealing to my responsibility. My identity, when the Other appeals to my responsibility, is *the-one-called-to-be-responsible*. I cannot turn away from the Other. I am there. This means I cannot turn away from myself as the one called. Levinas says I am trapped in my skin, too tight for comfort. The sensibility of my skin, my eyes, ears, nose, tongue cannot help but receive the revelation of the Other's calling me to be responsible. Regardless of what I decide to do, I am there and I must respond, *"Here I am."*

The first expression to me is the Other's presence and neediness before any talking. Levinas says that the face is the first word. The face of the Other says without opening its mouth, "Do not do violence to me. Serve my needs." My saying "Here I am" is the second word. I need not open my mouth. My presence says "Here I am. I have heard and have been touched by you." I may choose to responsibly respond, to be generous, or to be mean and nasty. But I cannot choose the occurrence of the original word of the Other, "Here I am, be responsible." Nor can I choose the occurrence of my saying "Here I am, I have heard your call." I can and often do respond with my *said*. For example, I make multiple rationalizations for not acting responsibly. I claim the other is undeserving. I bow out due to prior obligations. I demand my own equality and insist the other serve my neediness. The *said* speaks the language of equality, of my rights and chosen responsibilities. *Saying* speaks the language of inequality, of my responsibilities to the Other coming before my rights.

This distinction between the *said* and *saying* is especially important for therapists. My friend and longtime colleague here at Seattle University, Steen Halling, wrote over twenty years ago in an extraordinary and pioneering article, "Implications of Levinas' *Totality and Infinity* for Therapy":

> The therapy situation may be one place where we can hope for genuine discourse to take place, at least occasionally, and where the hours of rhetoric may be interrupted by moments of conversation. The hope resides not in the wisdom and cleverness of the therapist, but in the fact that we are in the presence of someone who may dispossess us of our understanding, our comprehension, and allow us to hear and to speak. (1975, p. 221)

Before the end of this section, I must throw in a couple of lines from Emily Dickinson's poem 1212 that haunt me every time I think about this distinction between *saying* and the *said*.

> A word is dead
> when it is said,
> some say.
> I say it begins to live
> that day.

Enough said here. Levinas offers us these compelling concepts. There are many more. I find these compelling when I consider a psychology that would be a *psukhology* of responsibility: the study of the desire of the psukhe to hear the ethical call of the Other compelling me to question my legitimate but ego-centered efforts for need fulfillment and to be of service to the Other.

But before we can describe this call of the Other, this power of the weak over me, we must describe the experience of power as power, and then the experience of weakness as weakness.

PART II

The Egology of Power and Weakness

CHAPTER THREE

Power and the Power of Power

A few years back, the graduates of twenty years earlier invited me with other faculty to their reunion. Many had gone for post-graduate studies in law, medicine, education, engineering, some psychology. Most had started working in professions immediately after receiving their B.A.s. Some had only "jobs," looking yet to find their "careers." Some had followed what they considered their "vocation," some had gotten "positions," some were "specializing," a few were in "trades," one claimed a "legitimate racket," another was in, what still puzzles me, "the consulting game."

Although they had not officially honored him "the most likely to succeed," Gordan[1] had been remembered as the one who "could have it all." No one had considered Gordan their best friend, but everyone liked him. While he himself did not come to the reunion, many stories of him did. Although no one had kept in close contact with him, nearly everyone had heard of his various accomplishments. He was wealthy, bright, handsome, charming, admired, envied, not openly criticized by anyone, but still a puzzle. He was ambitious and had become highly successful. He had risen to a position of power in an international corporation. His classmates knew twenty years earlier that he wanted it all, that he could have it all, and now he did.

To put it in the language of this book, Gordan's intelligence gave him the knowledge of understanding. His energetic effort reached success in every project he set out to do, and he enjoyed the rewards of his success with delight. As far as any of his classmates knew, there were no surprising and ironic twists of fate in his story. A spouse of an alumnus said she thought he sounded boring, but those who knew him rejected that conclu-

---

1. Gordan is not his real name. As in some of the other examples I have changed a few facts to make the example work.

59

sion, although some thought him a bit distant. It was said that he now lived an interesting life much of the time in far-off enchanting countries. I wondered myself why he came to my mind as I wrote about the paradoxes of power and weakness. I know of no dramatic paradox in Gordan's life. So why do I introduce this chapter with the story of Gordan? My cautious answer: because I remember his confident ambition, his unfaltering success, and incessantly being pleased with himself as what I now call *cynical*. Perhaps it's my cynicism that suspects his cynicism. Nobody called his ambition cynical when we knew him on campus, nor did anyone at the reunion. He was never nasty or critical of others. He simply knew the ways of human behavior were fraught with deceit, manipulation, and self-indulgence, and he took those into account when he dealt with others. His classmates called him a "smart cookie," never naive. He was successful because he did not automatically trust others. His contracts and agreements were based on guarantees. No one called him cynical, only intelligent and successful, ambitious for power. One can't argue with his success. Let me, then, for the time being, drop the label of cynicism for Gordan and for this chapter on power. Gordan was smart, successful, and comfortable. He fit our image of a powerful person.

Our collective cultural logic works like this: *we accomplish self-identity by accumulating personal individual power*. From the point of view of the self, to gain power is to stake out boundaries and define the qualities that distinguish who the self is and who it is not. Gordan owned his identity. He knew who he was, acted out his plans, and deeply enjoyed himself. The relationship between his identity and his power seems obvious.

PHENOMENOLOGICAL METHOD: DISCLOSING AND DECLARING

We need this chapter on power and the power of power because, while power seems so obvious, it is deceptively ambiguous and psukhologically paradoxical. To penetrate power's ambiguity, we must first carefully lay out its obvious characteristics. This requires a phenomenological description, an unbiased disclosure of the phenomenon as it shows itself. We need this unbiased description of *power as powerful* for a background against which a psukhology of the paradoxical, of the *weakness of power*, can be contrasted. Let me first say how I will describe the relationship of power to its owner, and then describe it.

The task of phenomenological description is to make explicit that which is experienced at a more implicit level. Our reflection and description of personal power should state clearly what may be obvious to all: power empowers. I will begin with this assumption of obviousness. I will *disclose* by reflecting on what is shown to my observation. This disclosure is a pointing of my consciousness toward what can be known by me, what is evident to me. I must assume that anyone who would attend to what is evident to me could also disclose this knowledge. My method of description will be to simply *declare*, to state how that which is disclosed by my observation is there. I will use declarative sentences from the point of view of the "objective" and general "we," such as, "We are powerful when we use and increase our power."

This *disclosure* and *declaration* about power will be an egological reflection and description, a study of the individual ego defining, using, and enjoying power. This might seem like "macho phenomenology." No need for modesty. We are educated in the age of Super-Enlightenment, in which the natural and social sciences have given us the confidence that we can *know* how things work, we can *act* with success, and we can *feel* satisfaction generally whenever and however we want. So we can *disclose* and *declare* what shows itself to our sophisticated perception and description. This is not personally "macho," since "we" know that anyone educated in this age of Super-Enlightenment can and likely does *know, act,* and *feel* like us. This may be culturally macho. Yes, the individual is powerful. But this power is democratically available to anyone.

I am going to use, now and then in this chapter, masculine pronouns. This is not meant to claim that men are more powerful than women. However, men have too often assumed they are more powerful, and in a later chapter I will show how this assumption can be seen as the basis for their paradoxical weakness. Since this chapter on power is a preparation for the later chapter describing the weakness of power, I hope I can use this well-challenged masculine claim of power without offending anyone. I have tried to avoid sentence structures calling for gender pronouns in order to avoid that offensive style. But when I do, my use of the masculine pronouns is meant to indicate a bit of irony about the masculine assumption of power. Gordan will be the man my pronouns are meant to refer to.

POWER AND THE POWER OF POWER
AT THREE PSYCHOLOGICAL LEVELS

What is psychological (egological) power? *Power* is the freedom of the ego to *know*, to *act*, and to *feel* the benefits of that knowledge and action.

Power at the *cognitive* level is *intelligence*: perceptive and rational. Knowledge gives us power to *understand*.

Power at the *behavioral* level is *exerting effort*: decisive and determined with energy. Acting with effort uses power to *develop skills*.

Power at the *affective* level is *satisfaction*, possessing goods and fulfilling needs. Feeling our needs satisfied provides us the ultimate power, *enjoyment* in possessing and consuming .

What is the power of power? *Intelligence, effort,* and *satisfaction* are powerful. They also provide the basis for making the ego even more powerful. The power of these forms of power lies in actualizing these powers as habits of knowing, acting, and feeling in order to gain more power.

At the cognitive level, the power of *intelligence* growing in *understanding* the complex situation of the ego, especially its basic needs, and comprehending the social and material resources to meet those needs, gives the ego the power to *make good judgments* and *right choices.*

At the behavioral level, the power of *effort* in *developing skills* gives the ego the power *to be successful,* to extend the ego's opportunities to know more and to act with greater skill.

At the affective level, the power of *satisfaction* increases the ego's *contentment* in consuming in order *to enjoy life* and *achieve happiness.*

The ego has a natural tendency not only for self-preservation (maintaining its existence), but also for self-development (expanding its existence). To expand and refine one's existence is simply to become more powerful. A powerful *individual identity,* the goal of modernity, strives to make good judgments and right choices, to succeed in its chosen actions, and to enjoy personal happiness.

Although this analysis discloses and declares the essence of power for individual identity, we must indicate that individuals are always immersed in the highly complex web of institutional structures and processes and the enormous forces of social power. In society, power rests in networks of routinized behavior of organized people. Individual power is gained by the possible and actual access to and use of these social structures to bring about or resist change. Hedrick Smith says in his book, *The Power Game,* describing the workings of politics in Washington, D.C., "Power is the ability to make something happen or to keep it from happening. It can spring from tactical ingenuity and jugular timing, or simply from knowing more than anyone else at the critical moment of decision" (1988, p. xxi). He explains that the most important knowledge is of *who* and *how* the powerful wield their power. Although the intention of this chapter is not to describe such "jugular" power of politics, this two-sentence description of Smith can be used as a model for the ways any ego exercises power, in sometimes lesser degrees, in its relationship with the surrounding world and especially with other selves in society.

The power of our individual identity does not pop into existence over night, as it does in our fantasies. The identity of the individual is gained over time through the recurrent experiences of its individual powers. The development of identity, at the cognitive level, is in the remembered and repeated themes in *understanding* through perception, thought, and choices: "I recall situations like this, and how I chose some successful and some unsuccessful courses of action. I am what I remember, and I will be what I plan." The ego knows itself from the past and anticipates its future. It learns by understanding itself and its situation.

At the behavioral level, individual identity is the set of skills developed by recurrent effort to succeed: "I kept trying until I got better and succeeded. I am and will be what I accomplish." The ego identifies itself by its experiences of perseverance and endurance in its successful behavior and overcoming failures.

Finally, at the affective level, identity is nourished by recurrent joy in the satisfaction of needs, and in overcoming the trials and tribulations that challenge that joy: "I've worked hard, taken the bad with the good, and deserve what I enjoy." The powerful individual, like Gordan, identifies himself by his ongoing contentment.

Let us more explicitly describe these means of power.

Cognitive Power: Intelligence for Understanding

Power, as an egological event of knowing, is achieved by clear *understanding* in order to make *good judgments* and *right choices*. "Knowledge is power," says the cliché. Naiveté is weak. Understanding the temporal, spatial, social, and personal circumstances of the given situation, and what role the ego can play, is the first condition of power. We make good judgments by comparing and contrasting our conditions with those of others, either immediately perceived or imagined. On the basis of these judgments, we can choose right behavior.

Not all knowledge is powerful, only that knowledge that *understands*, that which "stands under" and supports our potential or actual judgments and choices. Choice is the end and proof of the power of understanding. Having facts does not make a person powerful. In this age of the explosion of knowledge and the easy access to it, we tend to define knowledge too exclusively as the factual (scientific) description of an objective world and the technological skills to extract utility from this world. However, the detached observer, the possessor of factual knowledge, cut off from an awareness of any need and use for that knowledge, is not powerful. The knowledgeable person is powerful when intentions to connect needs with the available conditions inspires an understanding that allows choosing to act. In short, knowledge is powerful when it *motivates*.

Self-development books are exercises in motivational inducement. To motivate ourselves, these books tell us, we must first understand our needs and abilities. Secondly, we must understand the goods as rewards in our situation and the available access to these goods as satisfying those needs. And finally, we need to understand the power of other individuals and social structures that can help or hinder us. We need to then make judgments about what to choose. When it is said that "knowledge is power," it means that the person has a clear understanding of himself and the relevant conditions of the situation, especially the significant people, giving him greater freedom to make good judgments and right choices. People who are good judges of others make fewer mistakes in their deliberate choices. Their motives are placed firmly on clear understanding, just as their choices depend on strong motives. Clear understanding strengthens the possibility of, but does not guarantee, making good judgments and choices.

Powerful individuals do more than know what they want. They want it with a determination to act. They actually *choose* what they know and want. They are in control of their motives. Powerful people know that their motives cannot be mere wishes. Wishes are like puffed-up balloons, maybe filled with the passion of *wants*, but too safely secured inside us away from the risks of a dangerous environment. When wishes meet the sharp edges of reality, they get punctured, deflate our wants, and leave only a sagging memory. Wishes are too detached from the possible consequences of our actions to be called motives. Wishes are safe, but they are not powerful enough to motivate. Wishes can be turned into motives. Dreaming is not necessarily wasteful. But only motives that ground choices, motives that have been chosen, can give us power.

Just as wishes are not powerful, so excuses are even less powerful. Powerful individuals do not avoid responsibility by detaching themselves from their motives, claiming those motives were physical or social causes of the behavior independent of choices. They do not say, "My urges made me do it," or, "There is nothing else I can do; I have no choice." Motives are for them not causes. The forces of our physical, chemical, biological nature are causes, but motives are not. Physical forces occur without responsible free choice. They may have *might* or *force* to move us, but causes are not powerful in the sense we are using as the freedom to exercise one's will. Powerful people take full ownership of their motives. Motives, meanings that understand (stand under) our judgments and choices, are the very ground for those choices, precisely because we choose our motives. There can be no choice without motives, and no motives without choices. The relationship between motives and choices is not one of causality; it is dialectical. One does not *cause* the other. Motives provide the basis for choices, but the person must choose the intention to make that meaning a real motive.

We may have wishes and urges, but until they are chosen to be the grounds for our action, they remain merely wishes and urges. Physical forces act upon us, but until we understand these forces, and then own up to our choices, not excusing them as caused by those forces, we do not exercise real power in our lives.

Paul Ricoeur's classic book, *Freedom and Nature: The Voluntary and Involuntary* (1966), gives a description of the paradox of the dialectical relationship of motives and choices mutually supporting each other. He says,

> Thus the relation is reciprocal: the motive cannot serve as the basis for a decision unless a will bases itself on it. It determines the will only as the will determines itself (p. 67)

This description of how we choose our motives is not a claim that all choices are consciously reflected on. Most of our choices occur at the pre-conscious and predeliberate level. I do not wish to unpack all the psychological and philosophical arguments about conscious and unconscious, free and determined, motivation. On the one hand, Sigmund Freud tried to reduce us to automatons by exaggerating the power of unconscious (mechanical) motivation arising out of the id. On the other hand, Jean-Paul Sartre tried to raise us up to gods by exaggerating our freedom to know and control our motives. He called any claim to unconscious motivation "bad faith." Maurice Merleau-Ponty (1962, 1963) gives the most penetrating philosophical description of the ambiguity of the lived body knowing its world at both the pre-conscious and conscious levels. Perception consists in living the meanings of the world in the here and now. Reflection is founded on perceptual meanings and it abstracts those meanings out of concrete situations.

These philosophical conflicts and resolutions are important to maintain an abstract understanding of human power and motive. But the concrete experiences in daily life of our own power and our judgments of the power of others weigh heavily on some of us, while others could care less. For some, there is great motivation for personal power, to be on top of the situation. Uncertainty is unacceptable for them.

The extreme *ambition* of the power of power wants to achieve more than understanding in order to choose action. The word *ambition* comes from the Latin *ambi-* ("around, both or all directions") + *agere* ("to drive, to go"). The ambitious Romans went around seeking knowledge of others, manipulating votes to be successful in positions of power. The ambitious individual will determine to *comprehend* the situation to assure their choices will be perfectly *right*. The word *comprehend* comes from *com-* ("together, totally") + *-prehendere* ("to grasp, seize, embrace, include"). To comprehend is to totally grasp, to know exhaustively. The person seeking certitude is ambitious to fully understand, to reach out and hold totally the meanings of the situation. With total comprehension, judgments are guaranteed to be correct, with no mistakes, no errors from surprising conditions. With correct judgments, the person's choices would be absolutely right. He need not trust. Only the naive trust. The ambitious assure themselves of their *enlightenment* and are unhappy with any uncertainty. Gordan sought certainty to guarantee his judgments and choices.

Behavioral Power: Exerted Effort for Success

Power, as an egological event of action, *exerts effort* in order to *accomplish tasks* and *develop skills* for *success*. Success is the end and proof of effort. On this second behavioral level, the power of acting is being successful. "You can't argue with success," say those who are successful. We do not automatically succeed by some powerful motive jump-starting our well-practiced capabilities. Our intentions to act do not *move* our abilities. Natural talents and acquired habits, lumped together under the term *capabilities*, provide only the ground for action. But action can succeed, can be made powerful, by pushing those capabilities beyond previous successes. We must exert enough effort on our talents and habits to accomplish whatever has motivated us. Just going through some routinized motion is not enough. Effort is a kind of courage combining *will* with *risk*. People with great potential often do not succeed because they take their capabilities for granted or, fearing failure, they do not exert effort. Powerful people push themselves with a determination to succeed.

Paul Ricoeur (1966) is helpful again in describing the will that exerts effort, pressing our capabilities to give us our notion of the power of success. "Motor intention is the power of willing. There can be no willing without ability, and in the same way there is no ability without the power of willing (motor intention or effort)" (p. 327). He argues that just as urges and wishes can become powerful motives only when chosen to provide the ground for a choice, so capabilities can only bring success when pushed by exerting effort. There is a dialectical relation between pushed capabilities and successful action, just as between choice and motives. They mutually generate one another. The forceful and sustained exertion of effort in action strengthens the possibility for, but does not guarantee, success. Effort is always a risk. The uncertainty of the future of effort marks the experience of time.

The extreme *ambition* of the *power of power* for many people is to achieve more than success. They are not happy to simply exert enough effort to develop skills for further success. They want to *control* (*contra-*

"against" + -rotulas "a roll"). Individuals who control regulate, restrain, manipulate, exercise a dominating influence over the situation. Their ambition for power urges controllers to totally take over the action. They do not trust. Only total control guarantees success for the ambitious. The one who controls the situation, like Gordan, would demand perfect success, pure efficiency, the highest productivity.

Affective Power: Satisfaction for Happiness

Power, as an egological event of feeling, is achieved by *fulfilling needs*. Possessing and consuming goods, in order to be *satisfied* with *enjoyment* and *happiness* is the end of power. Enjoyment is not just an added quality, a fringe benefit on top of fulfilled biological and psychological needs. Enjoyment is the end of action. It is the love of life. Levinas says enjoyment is the very pulsation of the I. Possessing and consuming goods brings enjoyment. Happiness is the end and proof of the satisfaction of needs. By satisfying a need, enjoyment is an experience of power. Pleasure in the imagination may be turned into a motive to action, but it remains weak like the balloons of wishes. Enjoyment, in the final fulfillment of the motive to satisfy wants, is the only power you can sink your teeth into.

From an Aristotelian point of view, we could say that power is only attained in enjoyment as the final cause. Power is only secured in the fulfilling of the motive, in the success of the action, which finally offers the enjoyment of satisfaction. Until the final enjoyment, the powers of knowing and of acting are only means. They are only the sources to this end of enjoyment. Happiness is the ultimate. Final power is the enjoyment of the satisfaction of needs. Satisfaction strengthens the possibility for, but does not guarantee, enjoyment. Satisfaction is only the fulfilling of the need. Enjoyment is a kind of *willing*, an accepting and embracing the gift of pleasure from the satisfied need. Enjoyment is the end of the power of need-satisfaction.

The extreme *ambition* of the *power of power* is to achieve more than enjoyment. The ambitious do more than take in and possess the benefits of their successes. They wish to *consume* (*con-* "intensive" + *-sumere* "to take up"). To consume is to totally ingest, to expend, to use up, to waste, to squander, to destroy. Powerful people wish to fully absorb the thing into themselves, with no leftovers. With total consummation, no access by others to their belongings can take place. For the ambitious, consuming is a social exercise of power. They may be generous, but on their terms. They do not trust. They do not want others feeding off of or taking advantage of the rewards of their success.

Putting the three levels (the cognitive, the behavioral, the affective) together, from the point of view of the ego establishing its identity, the individual says, "Here I am. Notice me. I understand my situation. See how I know my 'here.' I use my understanding to motivate myself to make choices. I exert effort to succeed and improve my abilities. I make my 'here.' I enjoy the satisfaction of my needs. I consume my 'here.' This is how I empower myself. I am the center of my knowledge, action, and feelings."

These rough descriptions are not exhaustive, but they are workable definitions of egological power, divided into the three orders, or moments of, (1) understanding to motivate judgments and choices, (2) accomplishing success with effort, and, (3) enjoying satisfied needs. These are the definitions of *what power is*, and the *power of power*. Now we need to look at *how power empowers itself*.

HOW POWER EMPOWERS POWER

Power is more than understanding, effort, and satisfaction. I have described how clear understanding supports good choices, effort brings success, satisfaction gives us enjoyment. These results allow power to increase power. The power of power builds power in different ways.

To eventually articulate a beginning of a psukhology of the paradoxical, I want to open up an egological description of five ways in which an individual exercises power: (1) *centering* on oneself, (2) *serving* others, (3) *cooperating* with others, (4) *competing* against others, and, (5) *exercising authority* for managing others in the administration of organizations. In each of these I will describe the means to power in the three orders of human intentionality: cognitive, behavioral, and affective. Although this outline form may get repetitious, describing the three intentionalities in the five ways of exercising power, yielding fifteen different items, I hope it will prepare the reader for later descriptions of the paradoxical.

Centering on the Self

Centering focuses on oneself, free from any concern about others. Power can be gained by developing our understanding, our exertion of effort, and our satisfaction of needs for the purpose of self-improvement. We can attend solely to our own needs, abilities, and anticipated satisfaction in order to gain power for ourselves to strive for what we want. For example, we read thought-provoking books to know ourselves better. We practice forms of meditation. We exercise to improve our health. We reward ourselves with gifts to feel good about ourselves.

However, there is a tension in centering, a tension that is the basis for self-empowerment. Reflecting on our own needs, directing our acts toward ourselves, and nourishing ourselves is self-rewarding and self-perpetuating; it tends to sustain itself, to feed itself. However, centering is hard to hold on to. We get distracted. We get tired. We get satiated. There is simultaneously a centripetal and a centrifugal tendency, a pull toward our center, and a pull to outside ourselves.

On the one hand, centering benefits our needs, and therefore reinforces the continuation of centering. Our needs tell us to attend to them. They are not merely lacks, or empty holes. Needs are hungers. They are motives (movers), and therefore the grounds for choices. Fulfilled needs are the grounds for further self-directed motives. The power of choice from our own understanding pushes us to deeper understanding. The success of our self-directed action urges us to continue this centering. The enjoyment of satisfying our needs draws us to satisfy ourselves even more. We tend to get caught up and absorbed in our centering. Self-centering is self-perpetuation.

On the other hand, sustained centering is vulnerable to weakening, to fatigue. The discipline required to center cannot always be kept. We need to practice centering. There is great demand against the power of the will to maintain focused understanding, effort in action, and satisfaction of needs. Various needs compete for our attention. Needs wax and wane because they are not objective lacks, but subjective wants. We can lose our center and get dissipated. Our bodily energies get exhausted. Other people and things pull us toward them, and away from ourselves.

Centering, as a *declaration of independence*, claims that we are the source of our power and deserve the exclusive benefit of that power. This focus often conflicts with our deep desire for relationships with others. We can never completely deny our dependence on others for knowledge, abilities, and goods, and we can never completely deny the needs of others demanding us to attend to them.

Yet, for periods of maintaining and building strength, we can resist distractions, exert effort against weakening our intentions, and turn from any concern for others. We can recommit focused attention to our own needs, abilities, and satisfaction. Through strong motivated centering, we egologically define ourselves, at least for the moment, by saying, "Here I am! Right now, I do not need others. I do not owe others. I find strength in myself, and know how to benefit from my own actions." The ego can claim its exclusive center in the three orders of intentionality: in knowing, by *self-reflecting*; in acting, by *self-directing*; in feeling, by *self-nourishing*:

Self-reflection centers power in knowing. We can fold back within our consciousness upon ourselves and review our motives and actions in the light of our needs. We disclose in reflection our own ignorance and become motivated to understand our needs, abilities, and the surrounding conditions of our situation. We know how much and how little we understand in order to motivate ourselves to get a better understanding. We sharpen our already acquired understanding of our motives, abilities, and enjoyments to further strengthen our choices.

Self-direction centers power in acting. We can motivate our own motivation, direct our own direction. Self-directing is more than self-control or self-containment. Self-control is negative. Self-directing is positive. It means driving oneself. As we move with success we disclose new options for more effort. Sustained effort in practice requires our attention to strive for success. When we become complacent with whatever level our successes and abilities, we are no longer motivated to improve. Finding ourselves weak, we can exert effort to train ourselves to become capable. Or we can judge ourselves to be strong, but not strong enough, and push to further strengthen and refine our capabilities to accomplish even greater success. Practicing to increase power is consistently pushing our abilities just beyond a previous level of success. Centering for self-direction increases the possibility of greater success.

Self-nourishment centers power in feeling. Because we anticipate our tendency to be distracted and to get tired, we nourish ourselves to maintain our own self-centering. We take care of ourselves by rewarding our hard work in study and in exercising our skills. Even while busy self-reflecting and self-directing, we anticipate the satisfaction of our needs. In the midst of enjoyment, we can be motivated by our satisfaction to try for even more satisfaction. We enjoy our satisfaction so much that we get unsatisfied with this level of satisfaction and anticipate greater enjoyment. We nourish our life by enjoying the satisfaction of our needs, and motivate ourselves to want even more satisfaction for more enjoyment, more nourishment. Since satisfaction fades, we nourish our lives by anticipating a state of dissatisfaction and motivating ourselves to exert effort to maintain and increase satisfaction.

Self-centering by self-reflection, self-direction, and self-nourishment empowers the self.

Serving Others

Serving is the use of power to benefit others. We turn from centering on ourselves and attend to their needs. Although, we assume, at least for the moment, that we have enough understanding, success, and even personal satisfaction to help others, our service increases our own knowledge, skills, and satisfaction. Serving others is an exercise of our power for the benefit of both those served and ourselves.

The power of serving has its own tension. It requires some self-denial. First, we must give up some of our own understanding of the other in order to listen to them describe their needs. Second, we give up some of the effort directed toward our own success in order to act for others. We have to drop our own projects. Third, we give up satisfaction of our own needs to provide for others. We have to postpone our own gratification. A careful balance must be maintained between self-denial for others and the self-benefit from this denial. If we deny too much, we develop resentment. If we benefit too much by using the neediness of others to practice our skills and ennoble our generosity, we feel guilty.

Recognizing our inability to fully understand the Other, our lack of skilled abilities, and our lack of confidence that we have satisfied their needs by our help is a learning experience. Serving others, even with our limited understanding, abilities, and satisfaction, refines and strengthens them. We especially gain a sense of personal worthiness. Frequently, people say that they get more out of serving others than they were able to give. This "more" is a sense of self-worth and self-esteem. I believe it was St. Augustine who told us of three kinds of happiness: *litus* is the happiness of satisfied needs; *beatus* is the happiness of knowing the good; and *felix* is the happiness of self-esteem. The self-esteem gained by serving others makes us more powerful.

As we serve another, we define our identity in the realm of power when we say, "Here I am! I have given up a bit of my self in order to help this person. But I have also gained something by sharpening my abilities and worth and I feel pretty good about myself."

We can serve others, in the order of knowing, by *teaching*; in the order of acting, by *helping*; and in the order of feeling, by *providing*:

Teaching is the power of serving, at the cognitive level of knowing. We give knowledge to others so they can make better choices. When they do not have a clear understanding of their own needs and abilities, institutional structures, or other social and environmental conditions, or even a clear anticipation of their own possible satisfaction, we can serve by disclosing to them these aspects of their life. Probably, our most common means of serving others is to give them directions about means and then motivate them to work. Others often know their needs and have the ability to act, but they lack some information necessary to carry out the action. Giving this information can push them into action. Our research on the needs of others, educating them about facts, and training their skills, in turn, improve our own understanding of these facts and skills, and therefore gives us a sense of self-esteem as a teacher. Every teacher admits they most fully learn material when they teach it to others.

Helping is the power of serving, at the behavioral level of acting, doing the task, either partially or wholly, for the good of others. Even with the knowledge of what to do, others are often unable to be successful. If we have taught them, and, for various reasons, they still cannot act, we may serve them by doing their work for them to help them avoid failure. Helping others, of course, improves not only our own skills, but also our sense of self-esteem as a *helper*.

Providing is the power of serving, at the affective level of feeling, giv-ing the needed goods to needy others for their enjoyment. Since the goods themselves are usually the desired end, to serve is often to simply give the goods without either teaching or helping the other. The proverb says, "When you give a man a fish, you have fed him for a day; when you teach him how to fish, you have fed him for a lifetime." Yet we know the limits of this proverb. People need nourishment now. Some cannot provide for themselves, and need us to get them the goods. We especially feel good about ourselves when we have satisfied others' needs with gifts.

We can easily recognize in our self-disclosure that teaching, helping, and providing for others contributes to our own power.

Cooperating

Cooperation means working together with others to achieve a common end. We can exercise power by exchanging power with another under an implicit or explicit contract for both the mutual sacrifice and mutual bene-fit of each. Cooperation is less an agreement to trade equal work, more a combining of power, founded on the condition that neither partner could succeed without the other. Alone, each is less likely to gain; together, both are more likely to benefit. The special feature of cooperation is an agree-ment of *reciprocity* that guarantees shared effort to assure fair cost and an agreement of reciprocity to assure fair benefit.

In cooperation, we attend to the needs of others as we attend to our own, and it is the very providing for the needs of others that provides for our own. We support others' supporting us, while they support us, so we can support them, and so forth. In cooperating, we not only give power to others and increase our own, just as we do in serving, but we also strengthen the partnership. We form a unique bond in cooperation. In serving others, certainly cooperation is necessary. But in principle, the bond is different. Each role has a relative independence of the other. The server does not need the served, and the served is not required to give back to the server. In cooperation, however, the partners recognize their needed bond, some common good beyond the benefit each could hope for on their own.

Tension exists between the two aspects of the necessary bond in cooperation: (1) the reciprocal sacrifice for each to succeed and (2) the anticipated reciprocal benefit each expects to gain.

Although there are often explicit rules to assure the reciprocity of this *social contract* for giving and getting, *trust* is necessary to maintain this tension. The word *trust* is etymologically related not only to the word *truce*, but even more closely to the powerful word *truss* "a support beam, that upon which the weight of the structure rests." It comes from the word *traust*, "firmness." We can see that it is a not-too-distant cousin to the word *true*.

Trust is often unguarded. Yet cooperation carries the safety feature of the implicit threat to get out of any contract if the other violates the trust. Partners in cooperation not only need each other and work together toward a common goal and a shared success, they implicitly say to each other, "I'm watching how much you give and get, and I can quit if you cheat." The power of cooperation rests on the possibility of the collapse of the truss. It is assumed that neither partner wants this collapse. For the most part, this implicit understanding is left unspoken and basically unguarded. The truss is trusted.

Although, partners usually hold their trust in private, a violated trust, or the threat of one, can be made public. A violated partner can turn to others, and even turn to some protective agency that guards contracts by law. We can threaten to announce or prosecute a violation of trust to keep the other partner cooperating. Third parties can be called for witness and protection. Ordinarily, third parties trust the trust between those cooperating and assume they will not have to intervene to assure the cooperation between the original partners. The opportunity to trust the cooperative efforts of partners serves third parties. Trust between partners serves the *common good* of the whole community. Everyone else can get on with their own business and not worry themselves with the business of other trusting, cooperative partners. Cooperation is very powerful for everyone.

There is often more *common good* to the community than this simple release of third parties from having to intervene in others' uncooperative conflicts. Cooperatives usually serve other others. Loving couples make good parents to children. Good families make good neighbors. Cooperative business partners produce beneficial products. Teamwork in sports entertains spectators and provides models for other forms of cooperation. Aligned governments serve their citizens and other governments.

Despite the general good of cooperation, we find alliances combining power in order to compete against other alliances. In the highly complex structures of our modern organized society, power seems to thrive on sophisticated maneuvers of cooperative pacts in order to compete against other pacts. The competition between cooperatives can become vicious. Often, innocent individuals get hurt by the fallout from competition between cooperating groups.

For the most part, if the tension between contributing and benefiting is maintained, cooperatives bring good results. In the midst of cooperating, we say, "Here I am! I am one who cooperates. I need your help, and you need mine. I'm giving as I'm getting, and we are both getting a common good."

We can cooperate with others, at the cognitive order of knowing, by *dialogue*; at the behavioral order of acting, by *collaborating*; and at the affective order of feeling, by *dividing goods*.

Dialogue involves an exchange of information, ideas, and affect with another for the broader and deeper knowledge of the partners and for the common stock of knowledge. Dialogue is the power of cooperation in the free flow of knowledge, especially for an understanding of the different perspectives of the partners. The word *dialogue* is made up of *dia-* ("across") + *legein* ("talk"). Open dialogue is the mutual exchange of descriptions of realities to form a common reality. In dialogue, we not only increase each one's information, we also modify the knowledge each originally held. We learn what the other knew, we become more aware of what we each previously knew, and we learn the connections between the two. From the dialogue between cooperative partners, the ego can also reach out to others in dialogue. The network of conversations becomes the arena for the development of society.

Collaboration is joining with another person to work for the benefit of each. We reciprocate help with another for the success of each and for the improvement of the common good. Collaboration is the power of cooperative management when the task requires more than our own strength, skill, or tools. Like dialogue, collaboration is more than an addition of two powers directed toward the same action. The bond between the partners has a value in itself, and it usually supports the bonds to third parties. Collaborating is more than the increase of vertical strength with two lifting. The horizontal combining of power to form cooperatives reaches out to others.

Dividing goods means giving away some goods in exchange for receiving other goods, for the mutual satisfaction of the needs of the cooperating partners. But exchanging goods can be more than satisfying individual needs. When we give away a gift, we give a bit of ourselves. When we receive, we thank the other for their generosity as well as for their gift. The mutual support of happiness is the power of good community.

Disclosing experiences of cooperation allows us to declare that dialoguing, collaborating, and dividing goods gives power to the ego.

Competing

Competition involves striving against another to gain a benefit awarded only to the winner. Essential to structural competition is the limit to the prize: it only goes to one competitor, in a win/lose situation. There is always risk. To be winners, there must be losers. We not only try to gain, we also try not to lose. To win we try to make the other lose.

There can be gradations of winning and losing (first prize, second prize, etc.), when there are more than two competitors. There can be gradations within a divided prize through structured proportions, the first winner getting the largest portion, the second place getting the second largest, and so on. The limits from these gradations are set either by the independently established structure of the situation, as in commerce where one makes more sales or money than others, or by a competition design mutually agreed upon by the competitors, as in athletic games.

Alphie Kohn makes the distinction, in "The Logic of Playing Dirty," from *No Contest: The Case against Competition* (1986), between "structural competition" and "intentional competition." "The former refers to a situation; the latter, to an attitude" (pp. 3–4). Some people develop a habit of intentional competition, desiring to vie against others even in the absence of a situation structured by a limit on the prize. They thrive on competition because of the great feeling of winning, of excluding the prize from others, of being better than the other. Many people avoid competition because of the fear of losing. Competition offers pleasure and pain.

In situations of real scarcity, competition is less a choice than a necessity. Unfulfilled needs bring intolerable suffering. Losers really lose. Competition can get vicious. When people are forced into vicious competition for scarce but needed goods, we judge that something is wrong with the system. There ought to be enough for all.

In situations of relative abundance, especially in organizationally and technologically advanced societies, many claim competition to have special power to benefit all competitors whether they win or lose. Competitors seek the Other's challenge to push their own effort to succeed in order to improve their abilities. More understanding, exertion of effort, and enjoyment of the reward become the claimed psychological and sociological value of being challenged by another. The prize is not the only prize. The gain of making the choice, improving the skill, even when we lose, is worth the risk of loss.

The challenge of competition can be made to serve the common good of the community because the competitors can offer the community better service and better products. Power that is not properly challenged, however, tends to transform that power into self-serving. Unchallenged power tends to cheat the community. It can turn vicious against a weak competitor and hurt a community member, thus hurting the whole community.

The tension in competition is between (1) enough effort to win by beating the Other and (2) enough cooperation between the competitors to keep the competition going. Rules keep the tension in the proper balance. Limits are placed on conduct. Competitors strive to outdo the Other, and yet keep the Other in the challenge. By placing limits on their own conduct, they can continue to vie with each other. *Fair play*, the equal advantage set by the structure, is necessary to maintain the competition that provides the possibility of a *better-than-equal share*, encompassing all or a greater amount of the prize. Personal energy is gained through this tension where the motive to win the *better-than-equal share* threatens the *fair play* necessary to maintain the challenge (Alfie Kohn, 1986, pp. 158–66). The competitor says, "Here I am! I'm vying against others for this limited prize and I'm risking losing. But this chance of winning and testing my skills is a challenge that makes me try harder. I am how I have been tested and what I have accomplished."

Competition in the order of knowing is *debating*; in the order of acting, competition is *contesting*; in the order of feeling, competition is *marketing* and *shopping*:

Debating challenges the knowledge of others and offers a competing description of reality in order to persuade their understanding. We want our challengers to change their minds and give up their previously held understanding, in order to accept ours. Sometimes we want them to choose our understanding to join us in a common effort. Debates can smooth out conflicts so that participants can enter into cooperation. When there is a genuine search for truth, we can lose the debate by being persuaded toward the other's argument and thus gain a clearer understanding of reality.

While there are many reasons people enter into debate, three of them may help this discussion:

1. If the debate is genuinely for the sake of arriving at the truth, then it is not structural competition with limited reward. It is *disinterested* competition. The competitors are not interested in winning, but in the truth. There is no scarcity when the prize is truth. Truth is available to all without anyone's losing when others gain. This competition gets to cooperation in which each benefits.

2. If the debate is a formal contest structured solely to challenge the argumentative abilities of the debaters, in which the goal is not the truth, but the refinement of skills and the status of winning an honorary or real prize, then it is not a competition for the ends, but for the means. This is a kind of *disinterested-interested* competition.

3. Most frequently, the debate is to win the hearts and minds of others, to persuade them to vote for, or buy from, or join in an alignment for the sake of some other goal. Many people debate or argue simply to seek the power of winning. This is *interested* competition.

Whatever the motives for debating, the challenger's arguments clarify our own thinking by offering new facts and theory and by demanding that we refine our own expression of the argument to make it clearer to both ourselves and the challenger.

Contesting aims at outperforming another through using developed skills. Skills tested against genuine challenges are more likely to be sharpened than those untested. The skill of the challenger sets an immediate standard against which we compare our own. Athletic events are good examples, and the foot race is the best. We immediately see how far we are ahead or behind the challenger. Political campaigns with ongoing polling and final vote counts are often taken to be clear contests. Sales receipts in the marketplace also provide good indicators of our position in the contest. Political and economic competition is intended to serve the choice of the voters and buyers, but we often suspect unlevel playing fields with poorly structured regulations for fair play.

When the competitors offer counteractions against the others' skills, when there is defense as well as offense, skills of resistance and evasion of defenses are sharpened. We also develop speed and other abilities in seeking the goal. We learn how to maneuver better when we try to block our competitor's maneuvers and outmaneuver him. Team sports and one-on-one offense and defense games are good examples. The negative campaigning in both political and economic contests include the effort to make the challenger a loser.

Marketing and *shopping* strives to get the best benefit for the least cost. Marketers seek profits; shoppers seek bargains. The competitors are the sellers and buyers. Ordinarily we think of economic competition between sellers. Sellers try to attract buyers by offering better products and services, or by competitively lowering prices. The *science* of advertising has advanced to such a level that the buyer responds not to competitive shopping, but to the persuasion of the appeals of the marketer.

Very often shopping becomes an effort to get the best value in order to display an advantage over other shoppers, friends, and acquaintances, as well as the seller. We talk about our shopping feats as a kind of contest with others. Explicitly, the challenger is claimed to be the seller, but, implicitly, the challengers are those to whom we are recounting our exploits. This is *conspicuous consumption*: the prize is not just the goods, but especially the recognition of winning a competition. Shopping seems to be the number one American pastime, and being the best shopper, getting the best bargain, is the number one American virtue.

In abundance, competition for goods expresses to others our refined and *expensive taste*. People acquire goods of quality to compete with others in the arena of elegance. We can develop better taste by competing with others in the quality of our consumption. Competition in the area of satisfying needs for enjoyment may benefit all by raising the quality of the goods. But it can distract competitors into shallow striving when the necessity of the goods is outweighed by the effort in consuming for ostentation.

In situations of scarcity, we should not call this competition for goods "shopping" or "conspicuous consumption." Where the goods are limited, yet needs must be satisfied, and everyone has essentially the same needs, then the gain of one brings threatening loss to others. This is called survival. These competitions for essential goods, for example, food or shelter, can get vicious. In such states of war, people often "play roles in which they no longer recognize themselves" (Levinas, 1961/1969, p. 21). And yet, in circumstances of extremity (holocausts in ethnic and class conflicts, economic depressions, natural disasters such as widespread droughts) there are examples of extraordinary self-sacrifice and generosity, alongside of vicious fighting and conspicuous consumption.

Exercising Authority

Members of a community (common citizens, employees, organizations for leisure or worship, etc.) invest power in an authority in order to consolidate their power to avoid harmful competition against each other and against other competing consolidations. To avoid chaos, they assign themselves as subordinates to a leader who is assigned to administer the community power. Subordinates must give up some rights of choice and satisfaction in the use of their power by handing it over to the authority to be used for the common good of the group. The authority then has rights others do not have. Reciprocally, their authority has obligations and responsibilities others do not have. The power of authority is for the service of those who gave up power to those in authority. Implicit in establishing management by authority is that organized power is more efficient than disorganized.

Management has the right and obligation to know and interpret the indicators of the needs of the community, to authorize plans, to set policies, enact regulations, judge and enforce compliance, inflict punishment, and give reward. Often there exists a division of these roles of authority, because there is a tension between two major functions of authority: being sensitive to the needs of the individuals in the group on the one hand, and efficiently managing activity to provide both good quality and high quantity of service, product, or benefit on the other. Consideration for the subordinates' needs shown by communicating, explaining policies, and promoting trust in the authority often conflicts with the other function of assuring productivity.

For the sake of efficiency, the authority does not seek a challenger (as in competition) or mutual sharing of power (as in cooperation) because authority wants exclusive rights to make decisions to direct the power of others. This exclusive exercise of power for the sake of power can then free that power to better guarantee its use for the desired ends of the community.

Investing authority in a single person, and dispersing power across limited areas in broadening layers down a hierarchy or chain of command is considered by many the most pragmatic use of organizational power. A hierarchical bureaucracy streamlines efficiency for the success and satisfaction of its ends. Power by hierarchical authority is most like a machine, in which the parts are guided by a central energy and toward a single goal. The other means of power outlined above (self-centering, serving, cooperating, competing) diffuse power in large organizations, and can guarantee less apparent success than can authority that places power over many people in the hands of one or a few. Someone needs to take charge and accept responsibility.

The *science of management* has become very sophisticated with new models guided by differences not only in efficiency, but also in gender, age, ethnicity, and a host of other factors. Cooperative sharing of power, horizontally rather than in a hierarchy of authority/subordinates, is being worked out in many systems.

The exercise of authority is, however, very vulnerable to abuse, because some subordinates too easily give up freedom and some superiors too ambitiously seek the power to exercise free control over those who give it up. But it is precisely this vulnerability, this buildup of power in one source, and the reduction of power among the many subordinate sources, that makes it efficient and attractive.

Implicit in the exercise of authority in management is not only centering (concentrating power in the self) and serving (choosing to work for the good of those under the authority of the self), but also cooperating (mutually agreeing to give and receive power and to exercise it justly), and some competing (challenging each other to follow the lines of the structure and fulfilling the jobs of each). The tension lies in maintaining all these ways in the use of power. This is the tension between freedom and responsibility. The leader says, "Here I am! I am leading the others to achieve a common goal. My identity is in having more rights, but also bearing more responsibility."

Authority at the cognitive level of knowing *evaluates and plans* for the good of the organization; at the behavioral level of acting it *manages* by directing behavior and containing costs; at the affective level of feeling it *distributes benefits* to the members for their contributions:

Evaluating and planning empowers an *authority* through knowing the common goal, the needs of the members, and the actions required to get the job done, and dispensing that knowledge to those engaged in separate parts. A central plan needs to guide the distribution of tasks among the worker. The knowledge of each individual subtask may be held by particular subordinates, likely experts in their area. But when the task is so complex that the overall plan must be focused and located in one person or unified group to free those under it to attend only to their own part, then an authority of knowledge must be established. Knowledge of the power of an organization consists in knowing who holds the pieces of knowledge and skills and deciding how they fit together. The powerful authority designs the plans and communicates them to the subordinates to motivate them to choose to work hard and be productive.

Managing exercises *authority* by coordinating and commanding the subordinates to carry out their particular part of the overall action, in the right place and at the right time. The subordinates must assume the person in authority commands their action in coordination with those in other parts and, of course, for their own good. The authority must assure the subordinates that the commands and directives to act fit the ordered actions of others. The responsibility to avoid breakdown rests in the power of the authority.

Distributing benefits gives the *authority* the power to decide who receives what and how much benefit from the combined effort of all. This is probably the area of the greatest responsibility. Subordinates can sometimes tolerate gaps in the leader's knowledge of the corporate structure and activity and glitches in orders, but never the unjust distribution of rewards. They can fill in needed understanding and correct mistakes in actions, but they depend upon the leader for the orderly distribution of goods.

CONCLUSION

So this is power, and the power of power. I make no claim to fully understanding these exercises of power, especially in the last arena of authority. Centering the self, serving others, cooperating with others, competing with others all seem relatively simple compared to the complexity of organizational behavior. We live in an age of massive and complex systems of organization. The social constructionists have been persuasive in their theories of the reduction of individuals to social products. But something is missing.

This chapter's *disclosing* and *declaring* the nature of power and the power of power comes from an egological point of view. The ego is the central character in this analysis of power. Sustaining itself, perpetuating itself, relating to others as means to the ends of its ambitions, these are the accomplishments of the ego. These bring it understanding, success, and happiness. The obvious power of power seems to admit only its opposite, the weakness of weakness. Any suggestion of a paradox where a weakness resides in the very nature of power, or of a power coming from weakness itself seems ludicrously self-contradictory.

CHAPTER FOUR

Weakness and the Weakness
of Weakness

In an off-campus bookstore, I recently ran into one of my students under a big sign, SELF-IMPROVEMENT. She was focused on one of the most popular of the many self-help books on the shelf. I was surprised to see her there. I thought I knew her well. She would graduate in another year with a 3.8 something GPA, and hoped to go on to graduate studies. She has many excellent qualifications: she writes well, speaks eloquently, gets high scores on exams. She has every reason to be confident of success in her ultimate plan to be a clinical psychologist working with teens caught in violent gangs and abusive homes. She had taken some business courses just in case she could not get into graduate school. Maybe I did not know her well. Maybe she did not know herself so well.

I asked her what she was doing with this *recovery from co-dependence* book. She said she needed some books on self-esteem, because she needed a surer sense of personal power. I made a few remarks about her academic skills and my confidence in her future in graduate school and in helping people with painful problems. She said she felt like an imposter. In comparison, most of her family and friends seemed so much in charge of their lives. I expressed my surprise and expectation that she would not only get in and finish graduate studies, but also establish a career as a therapist, and be very good at it.

My assurances did not seem to convince her. She kept looking through the books; so I looked with her. The subtitles were remarkably similar: "How to Empower Yourself," "Step by Step Process to Unlock Your Strengths," "Pathways to Self-Assertive Behavior," "50 Ways to Self-Love," "How to Sell Others on Your Abilities," "Release the Force within You." These books appeal to our insecurities in this frantically competitive world of individual achievement and recognition, and they promise

so much. There is a self-perpetuating vicious circle here: the more we succeed, helped by reading books and magazines named *self-something*, the
more we feel insecure in comparison to others, and therefore the more we
need self-improvement tips.

Gary Greenberg in his book, *The Self on the Shelf: Recovery Books and the
Good Life* (1994), shows how the self-help recovery books are founded on
an assumption of nihilism. Since it is "inherent in modernity's understanding of the self as a sovereign sole author of its own story, . . . there are
no distinctions independent of the sovereign and isolated self ruptured
from others" (pp. 7–8). With this definition of *nihilism* as "no distinctions,"
Greenberg points out that,

> the absence or insignificance of distinctions other than those aris-
> ing out of the reader's [of these books] authority (understood as
> that which makes her feel "okay" about herself). (p. 188)

Our basis for "feeling okay about ourselves" is founded on ground so thin
we try to shore it up with more isolating efforts. Our obsession with independent individualism has left us insecure and frantic to protect ourselves
against the invasion by others into our psyches. I remembered the question of a foreign graduate student,

> Why do Americans think they need to become *more* independent
> of each other? It seems to make them *more* insecure, and there-
> fore *more* assertive. They are like frightened, lost children.

Should psychology be blamed for creating this self-defeating dialectic between insecurity and assertiveness, or only for cashing in on it? Or,
with Madison Avenue's and television's exhibitionism of the rich and
famous as models on the one hand, and of our self-criticism as losers on
the other, is psychology inattentively collaborating in making insecure
psyches, each weakening under the weight of a *too heavy self*, or better, *too
much ego*? Philip Cushman's article, "Why the Self Is Empty: Toward a
Historically Situated Psychology" (1990), places much of the responsibility on both contemporary psychotherapy and advertising for contributing
to the emptiness of self and simultaneously benefiting from this sorry
state by offering us the opportunity to heal our empty selves.

Toqueville, who visited us in the 1830s, said of Americans, they are
caught in

> restlessness in the midst of prosperity. . . . "[T]hey never stop
> thinking of the good things they have not got." . . . This restless-
> ness and sadness in pursuit of the good life is intensified, . . . by
> "the competition of all." (Bellah et al., 1985, p. 117)

Since Toqueville's visit, insecurity and defensiveness concerning identity has, in many cases, gotten much worse. The security of belonging to family, neighborhood, religious group, and citizenship has waned. Individual self-identity has taken on almost supreme importance and simultaneously become more fragile.

Let me return to the student in the bookstore. She was not looking for power in those self-improvement books; maybe she was searching for the weaknesses she was sure were in her personality but was keeping herself from admitting. From the public press and fictional television, the stories of failure and awful consequences that befall those who fail are meant to frighten her, and they do. Although she had not failed, she knew she had weaknesses; she felt like an imposter; she must find and get rid of her weaknesses and live up to an image. She suspected she did not possess the right stuff to challenge the field of tough competitors in her life ahead. Even though she was told by teachers, family, and employers that she could "make it," she felt she could not really trust their judgments. They favored her too much; she had perhaps unconsciously deceived them. Admissions committees and personnel officers, on the other hand, were neither nice, nor deceivable. They chose on the basis of profiles of abilities based on hard facts. They played *hard ball*. They searched for weaknesses, found them, and could destroy you.

I will describe the obvious characteristics of weakness, as I described obvious power in chapter 3. Weaknesses are liabilities, they drag us down, they are unwanted. We try to rid ourselves of weaknesses. We ought to be able to get rid of them because, after all, common wisdom tells us that they are due to our weakness. That is, they are the result of our weak will, and, with the exertion of our strong will, we can rid ourselves of weakness. Although our weaknesses are our fault, this is a blessing, because effort can make us powerful. Everyone is embarrassed by their weaknesses and strives to get rid of them. My student was alone, in a bookstore, somewhat late at night. I think she was *surreptitiously* looking at pulp self-improvement books. I was surprised to see her there, and she was surprised by my finding her there. Yet, as I thought about it, I should not have been surprised to find her there. She, like all of us, is under pressure to know herself, especially her weaknesses.

Certainly, we know the difference between weaknesses that have been forced on us by nature or the power of others, and those due to our weak will. We know the difference between *being weakened* and *being weak*, just as every child knows the difference between *accident* and *on purpose*. Yet, in comparing ourselves with others, we may not distinguish the two so easily. Social psychologists have lots of data to show that we publicly tend to attribute *dispositions of weakness* to those who fail, and, for the same failures in ourselves, we attribute the *situation* as the cause of our *being weakened*.

> When the actor has failed, . . . the observer will be inclined to invoke dispositions of the actor, whereas the actor will be inclined to invoke situational opportunities and constraints. (Ross and Nisbett, 1991, p. 140)

In other words, we blame others for their failures, and excuse ourselves for our failures; we also claim our own success, and attribute others' successes to outside conditions.

Not uncommonly, we use false humility to gain power. We fake humility by too smoothly telling others of our weaknesses. When we too publicly point out our own faults, we are speaking as if the self, the accused weak one, were distinct from the self, the accusing one. An apology is too often used to restore a damaged self-image, rather than to restore a broken relationship. All this hiding and excusing serves to defend our egos.

We think others' weaknesses, however, are not so hidden from us. While others cannot so cleverly disguise their weaknesses from us, we think we can disguise our own from them. We consider ourselves quite observant and can point out others' weaknesses, while we are also quite self-reflective and apologize only for those weaknesses we wish to display in order to seem modest. The weaknesses of others are obvious and are obviously the fault of those who have them.

In chapter 5, I discuss the paradoxical self-deception of being an *unseen seer*, the one who is convinced of her ability to hide her own weaknesses, and, at the same time, be highly perceptive of the weaknesses of others. In this chapter, I will stay within the phenomenological mode of observing and describing the "obvious," at least to the ego.

PHENOMENOLOGICAL METHOD: EXPOSING AND ACCUSING

Before I get into the description of weakness and how weakness weakens itself, I'll quickly review my justification for choosing this tricky phenomenological method. How do I justify the particular manner of reflecting on and describing without prejudice the phenomenon given to my observation, the human weakness that is obvious to any ego? To avoid the false sense of humility I wrote about above, that is, defending by too easily apologizing, I will not reflect on and describe my own weakness. To avoid being uncharitable to any specific person, I will not reflect on and describe the weakness of a named other. My phenomenological reflection will be to *expose* the weakness of the singular other, the weak one, the one who represents general others, all weak ones, *they*. Having *exposed* the weaknesses of another by reflecting on her/his expressions of knowing, acting, and feeling, I will *accuse* this other of the weaknesses I expose with my observation.

Weaknesses are weak. They are not valuationally neutral. The act of describing weakness is essentially an accusation. If I do not wish to accuse, then I should not observe and describe another's weakness. This *exposing* and *accusing* is a justifiable phenomenological method of description. The third-person singular pronoun will be used to refer to the accused, to clearly distinguish the other from us. From an egological point of view, the other is not like us.

Rather than use the first-person singular "I," I will use the first-person plural pronoun "we" to refer to us, the accusers, the ones who are observant and perceptive of others' weaknesses. Let me explain further the reason for transforming the "I" to "we." Blaming is not only used to accuse another. It is also used to seduce other others to join in the accusation in order to strengthen the original accuser's position. An accuser has to have confidence that her/his own weaknesses are hidden from others. Seducing others to join in accusing someone directs attention toward the accused, and away from any weaknesses of the accuser. For an egological methodology for phenomenologically describing the weakness of another person, therefore, I will use the plural "we," rather than risk using the singular "I," to hide myself from being seen as an accuser. To be an *unseen seer*, I must have *you others* on my side of this subjective seeing to make a "we" in this accusation of another person. This egological methodology is meant to protect against the exposure of my duplicity as the original *seer*, *exposer*, and *accuser*. To retain the mantle of objective observation, "we" are blaming, not just "I."

This is a tricky task, but not uncommon. It is used by many as an *objective* description, despite its *egological* bias. Editorial writers, talk-show hosts, standup comics, gossipers over the back fence, in bars, and in board rooms, although they do not explicitly claim the method of *phenomenology*, they have convinced themselves that they are *objective observers*, that is, they are revealers of what ought to be obvious to anyone who would be as observant as they. Because they consider themselves *perceptive*, highly observant seers, their looking *exposes* the weaknesses of others. Because they claim a fervent interest in *justice*, they are obligated to publicly *accuse* others of the weaknesses they have exposed.

I will underscore the *egological* bias of this phenomenology by using the feminine pronouns when referring to the weak one that I am exposing. I, as male, will play this stereotypical role of the *unseen seer*, too often the *voyeur.* I risk this irony in this chapter because in chapters 5 and 6 I will *be exposed* as an ego-centered male. I hope the reader accepts my irony.

Before I get started on this *phenomenological* description of weakness, I wish to explain one more time what role the analysis in this chapter plays in the larger analysis of the paradoxical. To more clearly get to the insight of how weakness, always weak, paradoxically provides the basis for its own power, we must reinforce our prejudice against weakness in order to assure ourselves that it is the weakness of the weak, not some newly discovered power, that provides them power.

WEAKNESS AND THE WEAKNESS OF WEAKNESS
AT THREE LEVELS

What is psychological (egological) weakness? Weakness is the lack of freedom of the ego to know, to act, and to feel the benefits of that knowledge and action.

Just as the word *power* carries a positive connotation, so the word *weakness* carries a negative one. Let me describe the weakness of the weak person, and how her very weakness weakens her in the three orders of intentionality: *knowing, acting,* and *feeling.*

Weakness is the lack of freedom to know, to act, and to feel the benefits of actions. In *exposing* and *accusing* the general other of her weakness, we remind ourselves of the distinction made between *being weak* and *being weakened.*

At the cognitive level, the weakness of *knowing* is *ignorance*, being unperceptive, insensitive, or irrational. This is distinguished from being weakened by some outside influence, for example, receiving the wrong information, being *mistaken* or *naive.*

At the behavioral level, the weakness of *acting* is *not exerting effort*, being lazy or cowardly. This is distinguished from being weakened by something other than the person's choice, for example, being disabled or restrained.

At the affective level, the weakness of *feeling* is *dissatisfaction*, having needs unfulfilled, or possessing the needed thing and still being discontent. This is distinguished from being weakened by some outside source, *denied*, refused goods for needs.

For the purposes of our analysis, we will not focus on the weakness of an individual because she is *weakened* by something other than her own personal powerlessness. Being weakened may be occasions for her to arouse herself out of her weakness, or to challenge the power that weakened her. But, since we want to expose weakness as the opposite of power gained by her intelligence, effort, and satisfaction, and, since we assume people can correct their internally influenced weaknesses, we will expose and accuse not *being weakened* but *being weak*.

Weakness exists as the person's powerlessness to do what she wants. In social activity between the powerful and the weak, weakness is the absence of willfulness to independently understand, exert effort, and fulfill needs. Her unwillingness adds the need of dependence on providers; she becomes a burden for others. Or, her lack of willfulness to protect herself makes her vulnerable to the abusive power of others.

The weak person has no stable identity, or she has a scattered identity. Her identity is *weak*. She does not really know herself. Her actions are based on fragile foundations. Her feelings are either dissatisfied, or, when she claims she experiences satisfaction, joy, even happiness, her feelings are shallow. The identity of the weak person is not a product of her own definition. She does not deliberately choose a weak character. But she indeliberately allows herself to become weak. Her identity is a set of labels assigned to her by others. Directly or indirectly, she is called dull or stupid, and, because she hides from herself, she perceives herself as perhaps confused and a little insecure, but mostly misunderstood. She is called lazy and cowardly, and sees herself as unfortunate and frightened. She is called either too sensitive or too apathetic, and sees herself as a suffering victim. While the powerful define and own their identity, the weak have their identity, their selfhood, mostly ascribed by others.

What is the weakness of weakness? While *ignorance, lack of effort*, and *dissatisfaction* are weak in contrast to the power of *intelligence, exertion of effort*, and *satisfaction* these weaknesses have further negative consequences. They are not only weak, they weaken the ego even more. The weakness of these weaknesses lies in their inability to provide understanding, accomplish tasks, and fulfill needs, all needed to gain power. Weakness, is more than the lack of power to gain or retain power. Weakness is not neutral; weakness weakens weakness.

At the level of knowing, the weakness of *ignorance* lies not only in the *absence of understanding*, but even more in risking *bad judgments* and *wrong choices*, setting the person up for darker ignorance, more vulnerable failure, and deeper dissatisfaction.

At the level of acting, the weakness of *not exerting effort* lies not only in the *absence of accomplishment*, but even more in risking *failure*, providing the conditions for further ignorance, failure, and dissatisfaction.

At the level of feeling, the weakness of *dissatisfaction* lies not only in the *absence of satisfaction*, but even more in risking *suffering*, conditioning further ignorance, failure, and dissatisfaction.

Cognitive Weakness: Ignorance for Bad Choices

From the point of view of the person needing to know her situation, weakness is ignorance or the lack of understanding, and thus increases the likelihood of *making wrong judgments* and *bad choices*. Ignorance is due to *ignoring*, being inattentive to the conditions of the situation, and unreflective about those conditions. A person's ignorance of the situation leaves her unable to provide the basis for correct and strong motivation. A person must know the situation in order to have the power of understanding to make good choices. She must know her needs and the skills to succeed, and she must anticipate the final reward of satisfaction in order to choose to act. Ignorance of these expresses the first level of weakness. Ignorance does not guarantee bad judgments and choices, but it surely limits the chances of making good ones. Luck or the intervention of others, in spite of her ignorance, may provide the person with the basis of judgments and choices that turn out to be good, but with no thanks to her power. The person who must depend on luck or benign intervention is weak.

A weak person seems to be unmotivated. She has little upon which to base her wishes and natural urges. When she does choose, it is usually out of shallow motives, and she usually fails or gets in trouble. When the bad things happen to her, she blames them on others or on bad luck. She cannot own up to the fact that her behavior and reasons lead her to make bad choices.

Behavioral Weakness: Lazy and Cowardly for Failure

From the point of view of the person needing to carry out action, weakness is laziness or cowardice, and thus increases the likelihood of *failure*. A person must have strong skills and must exert effort with those skills in order to succeed. Inability may be from a lack of experience and training. While the weak person may attribute this to bad luck or someone else's fault, we can accuse her of carelessness or indetermination. She may say that she has been weakened by some obstacle in reality. But others judge her to be weak in failing to take action to avoid the difficulty. This inability to anticipate problems and prepare for them expresses the second level of weakness. Laziness does not guarantee failure, but it certainly makes failure likely. Again, luck and generous help can save her, but this is not her power.

Affective Weakness: Dissatisfaction for Suffering

From the point of view of the person's needing to enjoy life, weakness is dissatisfaction because of discontent with what is given the person, and thus increases the likelihood of justified *suffering*. Lacking satisfaction by not receiving the needed goods, like food, can be distinguished from receiving the good but judging that it does not fulfill anticipated enjoyment. Both can bring suffering. A person must have needs filled in order to enjoy life. But we know that too many people who are denied are not willing to imagine and exert the effort to seek and find the goods, to work for them, and to satisfy their wants and enjoy them. Dissatisfaction that flows out of not being content with what is given, or not being motivated to go after what is wanted, expresses the third level of weakness. We can accuse persons of this kind of dissatisfaction. It does not guarantee suffering, but it certainly lessens the chances for enjoyment.

HOW WEAKNESS WEAKENS ITS WEAKNESS

I heard of a teacher who uses a pedagogical trick to teach students the experience of comparative weakness. She asks the students to line up according to how much power they think they have. They tend to crowd down at the back of the line. We all seek power, and tend to avoid weakness, yet, when we are asked to judge our own level of power, we compare ourselves to those above us. Psychologists call this concept *relative deprivation*. Many people consider themselves poor because they look to those who are richer rather to those who are poorer.

A reason for a person to judge herself as weaker than others may come from her tendency to avoid the responsibilities attached to power. Many consider themselves to be in positions of authority, but they feel that their power is diminished by either those above or those below in the hierarchy. A person seeks power to control others, and to fulfill needs, yet a person may seek weakness to free herself from obligations.

Although a person tends to judge weakness in negative terms, she finds within the very nature of her weakness the basis for some power. She wants to avoid being weak. Yet she may find a strength in her weakness. First of all, as already indicated, her weakness releases her from any responsibility associated with power. Secondly, she may find her weakness has a kind of power over others. People feel sorry for her and do her work or give her things. A *passive-aggressive* style is precisely the use of feigned or real weakness to manipulate others. Her *learned helplessness* could be a style used to get what she wants by taking advantage of others who have a style of learned helpfulness. A buzzword among psychologists is *codependency*. This is a reciprocal set of habits whereby one thrives on caring for another's weakness, and the other thrives on having their weakness taken care of.

These styles of manipulation through the use of weakness to exercise power could be called *powerful* rather than *weak*. Yet the weak person more or less falls into them. She discovers her weakness has power. She may live among other weak persons who feed each other's weaknesses. But she is weak because her only real alternative would be to pull herself together and develop a strong identity. Always on the edge of her life are the opportunities to empower herself. Sometimes she does. Usually she wastes her life avoiding reaching a real understanding of her situation, exerting efforts to succeed, and finding real joy in the satisfaction of her needs.

Let us return to the recognition that the weak person has available the possibility to find in society and in herself the power to change. Some people turn their lives around. A weak person has that same possibility to empower herself, despite her developed patterns of weakness. The power of power, described in chapter 3, does not happen naturally. It takes understanding, energy, and enjoyment. The powerful empower themselves by intelligence, effort, and satisfaction. The weak could also become powerful, but she hasn't. She does not so much choose decentering, but rather passively is decentered. We should use the passive voice in these descriptions.

I will outline five ways weakness weakens itself, which correspond in contrast to the five ways to increase power. They are:

1. *Being decentered* rather than centered
2. *Being useless* to others rather than serving
3. *Isolating oneself*, or *giving way* rather than cooperating
4. Being *incompetent* or *uncompetitive* rather than competing
5. Being *impotent* rather than exercising the authority empowered to her

Being Decentered

A person can lose power by not attending to her own needs. When a person's situation turns bad, she needs to *focus, get a hold of herself, take charge of her own life*. But the weak person has not developed the power to do so. Another word to describe this tendency to decenter would be to *dissipate*, which means to *scatter away*. In chapter 3, we described how individual abilities help the person gain a level of independence from others who are either providers or abusers. Here, we can show how she allows her power to be dissipated, to become weak and dependent on others to provide for her needs, and thus weakens herself further. Her weakness also makes her vulnerable to the misdeeds of others, which further weakens her. Decentering reduces or scatters her understanding, effort, and therefore satisfaction. When she is decentered, she does not exercise her power to comprehend herself, to control herself, and to find her own sources of satisfaction.

Being *decentered* (dissipated, scattered, unfocused), at the cognitive level, means being *distracted*; at the behavioral level, it is being *indifferent*; and, at the affective level, it is being *apathetic*.

Being distracted is the weakness of decentering by losing the focus of understanding. This is the major source of the person's ignorance. Remembering that the etymological root of *ignor-ant* comes from in-gnoscere, not-to know, which means to ignore, to disregard, we see that ignorance is due to distractions. Either by a lack of focus, or by an obsession with other ideas, or by an insensitivity to her situation, she ignores knowledge necessary to make good choices and weakens her possibility for the power to fulfill her needs.

Being indifferent is the weakness of decentering by being unwilling to energize effort toward her own good. She can weaken her abilities to work for success, and therefore make herself vulnerable to failure by not exerting effort. She may try to convince herself and others that she is motivated, but unless she pushes herself to attend to the job with focus and tenacity, she cannot accomplish her needs. If her imagined satisfaction of needs remain at the level of wishes, then she is empty of power due to her indifference.

Being apathetic is the weakness of decentering by being unwilling to imagine the success and rewards of effort or to enjoy the goods she has available to her. She weakens her satisfaction (increases her suffering) by not consenting to the conditions in which she finds herself. She deprives herself of those things she has at hand and could otherwise enjoy with imagination and effort.

Certainly, people are dissatisfied when they suffer deprivation brought about by circumstances beyond their control. We might even call this dissatisfaction with scarcity a kind of strength. But the weakness of weakness at the affective level is being *apathetic* (*a*- "without" + -*pathos* "feeling") even in the midst of the possibility for enjoyment. Psychological (egological) depression allows some deprivation to occupy the person's attention while neglecting the satisfaction of other needs available to her. I am tempted to say that apathy develops from a lack of gratitude. Gratitude is primarily the enjoyment of a gift given, and secondarily the expression of thanks.

Being Useless to Others Rather Than Serving

Uselessness is lacking power to serve the needs and abilities of others. Not only does the person not help others, she often burdens those she ought to serve. Too often this means she depends on still other Others to serve those she should be able to help. This often implies that she depends on the others to serve herself. She needs their service to guard her from advantage taken by still others who recognize her vulnerable weakness. The server who cannot serve becomes not only a burden to others, but also vulnerable to further weakening.

Service demands self-denial. If the weak person cannot perceive the needs of others and even her own needs, if her skills are not available for the tasks, if she is uncaring and apathetic, then she has no way to deny herself and retain power to carry out the tasks of service. When she does not practice working for others, then these skills weaken. When she cannot be of service to others who need her, she does not have the possibility of self-esteem based on serving others.

Being uninformative describes the weakness of serving, in the order of knowing. Uselessness in having and providing knowledge to others comes from being unperceptive of others' needs, or not understanding the situation to fulfill these needs, or being unable to instruct them about how to fulfill their needs. We can recognize in the weak person a kind of shallowness or lack of depth. When we say that one lacks depth, we mean that the person cannot see far. This does not mean that she is of lower intelligence or has near-sightedness. She does not want to open the eyes of her eyes because she is distracted by her own narrow interests, or lacks courage, or is simply lazy. She is not able to grasp the deeper needs of a situation. This inability to understand others reveals a shallowness that makes her likely to depend on others to provide the understanding of others' needs and abilities. Her ignorance weakens her ability to deepen her understanding, and to have the knowledge of self-worth.

Being unhelpful describes the weakness of serving in the order of acting. Being unuseful in serving others may not come from lacking the knowledge or skill. Her lack is likely because of her laziness. When she is careless and cowardly in helping, she expends useless power doing the wrong thing or the right thing in a shabby way. This weakness in helping others makes her become dependent on others to serve her, weakening herself even further and lowering her self-esteem.

Being unable to provide describes the weakness of serving, in the order of feeling. Being useless in serving others by not giving them what they need, especially compassion, may arise out of a lack of concern for those others. A useless person may be stingy even of her own feelings. Being unsupportive often occurs because the person is dissatisfied and therefore has nothing to give to others. When she gets enthusiastic about what she is doing, she can nourish others. But when she is herself un-self-nourished, she may be able to give needed things, but she cannot give of herself and therefore cannot really nourish others. Discovering she simply does not care about the well-being of others contributes to the lowest self-esteem.

Isolated from Others or Giving Way Rather Than Cooperating

A person can lose power by not contributing her fair share in any effort to gain a common end. When a person enters a cooperative arrangement, she is defined as a partner, in an explicit or implicit contract based on reciprocity of skills, effort, and fairness in the division of the reward. In cooperation, a potential partner to the person looks for help because the partner knows she cannot do it on her own. This potential partner is willing to contribute her part, knowing the person also cannot do it alone. The person is asked by this potential partner to give attention both to her own sacrifice and benefit and to the other's sacrifice and benefit. If the person is not able to contribute as a cooperating partner, because she is fearful of trusting, then she weakens any cooperation.

Sometimes one is so needy of being connected with another, and simultaneously so fearful of offending the partner, that she offers no needed power to the relationship. She offers no contributing understanding, no exertion of effort, no need for satisfaction. She compromises herself so much and gives over so much of her power to others that she has no power to give to the cooperative venture. She is gripped by a psychological paralysis that keeps her from entering into a joint effort.

Compromising, rather than cooperating, can either isolate the person from others by escaping behind excuses of ignorance or disinterest, or by abandoning her position of values simply to avoid conflict. When one simply does not exercise imagination to offer ideas for the cooperative effort, including how the partner can contribute, then she offers nothing to the partnership. When the weak person gives over her individual understanding, her facts and ideas, in order to connect with another for the sake of connecting rather than for the sake of contributing knowledge, and does not expect any reciprocity, then she has compromised herself and denied to herself the very knowledge available to her. When she shows her desperate need for a relationship because she cannot bear to be alone, then she exposes her weakness. Either way, she becomes a burden to that partner, and thus destroys the cooperative contract.

Accommodating, rather than collaborating, isolates or gives way in the mutual activity with others. When the person cannot contribute any effort to the task to be done, and merely gives herself over to the other's orders, then she is accommodating and essentially not cooperative. This makes her dependent upon the partner, and allows the partner either to abuse her passivity or to break off the relationship because she offers nothing. The accommodating person is vulnerable to manipulation by the power of another.

Relinquishing, rather than dividing goods, isolates or gives way in the distribution of goods. A weak person weakens herself by giving up the benefit achieved from a joint venture. She supposedly enters into cooperative ventures because she has needs to be satisfied. When the weak person gives up the benefits, her needs remain unfilled and she remains weak. The partner expects to share in a cooperative relationship. Mutual enjoyment is the great reward of cooperation. When the weak person does not accept this sharing, she makes the other take all the benefit. If the weak receives no goods, the partner is not able to receive the reward of cooperation. The partner gets the goods but loses the partnership.

Incompetent or Allowing Defeat Rather Than Competing

Backing off from challenging the efforts of the other competitor weakens the weak person by losing any power to win, and losing any chance to improve her skills by the other's challenge. Competition requires risk. Cowardice keeps her from risking. When she is unwilling to risk, she offers no challenge to the other. When she cannot challenge, she has no opportunity for the opposition to challenge her in return. When there is no challenge, she does not test truth, common growth, and shared happiness.

Conceding, rather than debating, shows incompetence in the discussions of differences. Allowing herself to be refuted in arguments the person weakens herself in a debate by not challenging the facts and ideas of the other. A debate demands careful thinking by means of speaking and of listening. A debate, remember, is not a double monologue, where one keeps quiet while the other speaks, does not really listen but only waits for the other to shut up, and only really attends to her own imagination of what she will say when she gets the chance. In a quarrel, combatants usually challenge the other with arguments not necessarily addressing the issue offered by the other. In a real debate, each attends to the other's points, and responds to those points. The weak person weakens herself by not listening, or by not framing a response, and therefore losing an ability to respond to the other's points. She is not able to test truth.

Quitting, rather than contesting, reveals incompetence in artificially structured or real contests of skill. A weak person weakens herself by not exerting effort and losing any advantage. The advantage in a contest of action is the lead position. The word *advantage* is from the French *avant*, "before or ahead." When a person is weak she is trapped in having to catch up, to follow the lead of the other who has the advantage. She is forced to be defensive. This position weakens any opportunity to set the shape and pace of the contest. She cannot challenge the other and cannot adequately receive any real challenge that would test and strengthen her abilities.

Losing out, rather than competing for benefits by searching for the best reward, reveals incompetence by allowing herself to be deprived. The weak person weakens herself by allowing the Other to take nourishing goods from her. When she competes with another for limited goods, she risks losing not only the reward, but also exposes her neediness. Her needs do not disappear when goods are not attained. Hunger remains. When she does not receive any goods, she makes herself vulnerable to losing more because she is ill-nourished. She does not test happiness that comes from the celebration of the reception of goodness with others.

Impotent Rather Than Exercising Authority

The inability to properly exercise power to work for the good of the organization is a serious weakness in a person placed in a position of authority. Lack of essential knowledge for decisive judgments and choices, cowardly and unenergetic action, and loss of fairness in the distribution of rewards and restrictions are the signs of impotence. Power is invested in an authority by subordinates because they trust the person to have an understanding of their needs and the structures and processes of the organization, to have the courage to make necessary and sometimes risky decisions, and to achieve fairness of results. When the person of authority lacks one or all of these, then that person is a weak authority. Either anarchy reigns or others assume power from the weak authority.

Being indecisive, rather than evaluating, planning, and making good judgments and choices, a weak person in authority shows impotence in the tasks of knowing. A vision of the purpose, direction, and results of any organization is essential for decision making. Being ignorant of needs and ways to fulfill them or foolish in making decisions based on wrong or inconclusive data weakens the power of the authority. A person in authority often has to make plans and decisions with less data than she would want. But the time for a decision comes from conditions independent of her readiness. Perhaps we could say that all decisions are relatively untimely. Yet decisions must be made. An indecisive authority lacks the self-confidence and courage to risk. The weak authority is not smart and is unwilling to risk a decision.

Being ineffectual, rather than efficient in managing, shows impotence in authority in the order of acting. Managing the behavior of subordinates to fit the behavior of others in the organization defines the second task of the authority. Being ineffectual or uncourageous in setting a direction and giving orders weakens the weak authority for administering power by not exerting the effort to demand that subordinates act in ways that benefit the good of the organization. The weak authority either cannot order a subordinate to carry out necessary behavior, or she gives the wrong orders because she is ignorant of the proper orders. The weak authority is often a coward.

Not being in control of benefits, rather than fairly distributing them, shows impotence in authority. Taking command of the rewards and restrictions of subordinates defines the third task of the effective leader. Not being in control of dividing the profits of success and not being in control of penalties for the misbehavior of those under her authority weakens her. Authority must experience the needs of the subordinates and meet those needs in a fair way. Either someone else has this control and the weak manager is unable to gain it as the authority, or she does not sense the importance of rewards and punishment claimed by the subordinates. The weak authority is unfair.

CONCLUSION

So this is weakness. It is weakness described by an egology. Since it is an egology, a view of the behavior from the point of view of the ego maintaining and perpetuating itself, it can only *expose* and *accuse* weakness in the other person. But exposing this very phenomenological method of exposing and accusing will be necessary to reveal the weakness of power and the power of weakness. This present chapter does not describe weakness by a *psukhology*, a study of the *psukhe*, or soul, inspired by the weakness of others, where the Other's weakness accuses the psukhe itself of violating the rights of others. It takes paradoxical thinking to have a *psukhology*. This chapter's "straight thinking" of *egology* serves the ego well, but it misses the infinite value of the Other.

I apologize to any who might have been offended by my use of the feminine pronouns when writing of weakness. I hope this deliberately ironic method reveals the arrogance of the egological approach, trying to give an objective view, but unable to do so precisely because it cannot police itself. The face of the Other calls biases into question. The ego, solely from its own perspective, in its own power, assumes an ego-centered view of its own power and the weakness of others. We now must make that radical Copernican revolution, inspired by the philosophy of

Levinas, that places the Other in the center of the self, the Other who calls the biases of the self into question. This is the fundamental insight of *psukhology*.

PART III

The Psukhology of
the Paradoxical

CHAPTER FIVE

The Weakness of Power

Martin, over the course of thirty years, rose from teller to president of a large commercial bank. He had been recruited a few times by executive headhunters, worked his way through three different banking companies, and climbed up the chain of command with each move. He was very good at the tasks at each level of authority. He gained not only more power, but, of course, much more money and prestige.

He quit last year after having been president for only three years. We have been friends since college in the early sixties. He took me to lunch a few months before leaving the bank, and told me that he couldn't take the weakened power he had risen to. He said:

> Basically I do two things at my desk: I fire middle managers, and I foreclose on large debtors. I had a choice years ago to either go for the power and money, or get out and do something more humane. I went for the power and money. It was exciting all the way. But I had been feeling uglier and uglier at that desk since I first sat in it three years ago. I don't even want to live in the city. Barb and I are moving to our place on the island. I'm getting out before I choke whatever small sense of decency I have left.

"Power corrupts, and absolute power corrupts absolutely." We often repeat Lord Acton's epigram like a mantra because it rings so true, so often, in so many settings: "Power corrupts." We catch more than a glimpse of the paradox of the weakness of power in power's ability to sabotage itself when we see that the power assigned to a political leader has corrupted her or his authority, the unfair practices of a businessperson has led customers and competitors to boycott and sue, the abusiveness of a parent has sabotaged her or his parenting, the oppressiveness of a spouse has wrecked the marriage, the harassment of a boss has undermined her or his management, the intolerance of a teacher has diluted the lesson, and so on. The accumulation of power in personal, political, economic realms is constantly vulnerable, not only to outside competing powers, but even more to its own corruption, its own self-subversion. Power collapses under its own weight.

Despite many examples from our own experiences, the weakness of power often eludes our reflective analysis, especially our logical and rational understanding. Because power is powerful, and defensive about its vulnerability, we are blind to its potential weakness. The phrase "power corrupts" springs to mind only after we have witnessed abuse. Power, weakened by its own power, disguises itself and accuses others of being the source of its weakness. The power of power is obvious and seductive. The weakness of power shows this seduction to be an illusion, an erroneous perception of reality. The apparent obviousness of the power of power deceives us and prevents us from penetrating the hidden reality of the weakness of power.

This paradox of the seduction and illusion of power has been a consistent theme in the history of literature and the literature of history. A former teacher described history as simply the stories of irony: the great successes of power turning on and destroying those captured by its promise. Religious storytellers and other artists continually speak of the weakness of power. Because power continues to seduce and deceive, it makes us forget this paradox. The weakness of power is usually dramatic, often surprising, sometimes shocking, because reason is so easily convinced by the power of power. Logical thinking consistently tries to overpower paradoxical inspiration. Egological analysis tries to overpower psukhological description. History, literature, philosophy, theology, and psychology urge us to recognize that that which is revealed simultaneously conceals, and yet points to what is hidden and contradicts the obvious. Power as power conceals from us power as weakness.

In order to describe the psychology of this elusive paradox, we shift into another phenomenological method. In chapters 3 and 4, the method was to describe the phenomena of power and weakness as they revealed themselves to us from the point of view of the obvious power of power and weakness of weakness: the paradigm of an ontology where the ego is the center of the self. In chapter 3, the attempted method was an *objective* reflection *disclosing* the obvious to a detached observer. What was disclosed was assumed to be universally true to every observer, so the description was a straightforward *declaration*. I used the first person plural pronoun "we," confident that the reader and everyone else would have to agree with this declarative description of the experience of power arising from unbiased reflection on the obvious.

PHENOMENOLOGICAL METHOD:
BEING EXPOSED AND CONFESSING

In chapter 4, the phenomenological method of reflection was to *expose* the weakness of the weak person. Since any observer knows the power lost by the weak person is recoverable if she would only summon up the courage and effort, we can allow ourselves to be judgmental about the weakness of the weak, and justify our *accusation*.

The method to be used in this present chapter on the weakness of power is to point to what is beyond the phenomenon of the power of power, and the phenomenon of the weakness of weakness, namely the weakness of power. In this chapter I describe what is *exposed* in me by the face of the Other who confronts my judgments, my manipulations, my addictions to my own needs: that the Other is beyond my comprehension, control, and consumption. I describe as much as possible the paradoxical, (*para-* "beyond" + *dokein* "to think,") beyond what appears to the ego when the ego takes itself to be the center of its power. Since the vulnerability of the face of the Other reveals my egocentric tendency to violate her vulnerability, the phenomenological method is to *be exposed* by her facing me. My admission, my owning up to my placing my rights before my responsibility to her, demands I use yet another phenomenological method of description, I *confess*. I use the first-person singular pronoun "I." I assume nothing about any specific or general other. I describe what is revealed to me by being *exposed* in this confrontation by the face of the Other. This method could be called *confessional phenomenology*.

Inspired by the insights of Levinas to reflect on the experiences of the face of the Other challenging my egocentrism, I state the thesis of this revelation: *power is paradoxically weak when it is ego-centered.* When I egologically locate both the source and benefit of my power exclusively in myself, when I claim my will to have its origin only from me, and my needs its primary beneficiary, then, confronted by the goodness of the Other, I am paradoxically weak. I am confronted with the revelation that my ego-centered power can be self-destructive. I am weak because I can sabotage my authentic source of power, the investment of power in me by the needs of others, and I can deny my deepest calling to exercise this power by responsible service to the needs of others.

Other-centered power, power invested in the self by the worthiness and neediness of the Other, *is responsibility.* Levinas's notion of the investiture of freedom by and for the Other (1961/1968, pp. 84–90; 1974/1981) is an extraordinary insight for psychology. Responsibility inspired by the Other's investment of freedom provides the self with its authentic existence. The word *existence* is from *ex-* ("outside") + *-sistere* ("to stand"). To *exist* is for the self to stand outside itself, to transcend the ego, to find its place beyond itself, to discover itself in being responsible to the Other. This discovery is not an isolated self-discovery. Alone, I tend toward ego-centrism. The face of the Other exposes my selfishness and reveals my true self as responsible to others.

How do I sabotage myself when I cling to myself? As an ego, I am self-centered, but, as a person, confronted by the vulnerability of the needs of others, I find myself fundamentally Other-centered. That is, I recognize that others are *infinitely* more than what I can know of them. They resist my *totalizing* them. They have an infinite dignity and worthiness independent of my judgments. Their dignity and worthiness confronts my egocentricity, and calls it into question. I do not have an equal option between serving ego-needs or serving the needs of the Other. The desire to serve the needs of others has a priority over the satisfaction of my own needs. I may convince myself that I have two equal choices, but the call to responsibility questions my self-service. I receive power from others as freedom invested in me by the call to responsibility from and for the Other's neediness. My ego-centered power is, therefore, destructive of my most fundamental self. It is my own power that weakens me when I misunderstand and misuse my power by centering it on myself.

Certainly, as an individual, I have the possibility and tendency to claim power to myself. My freedom can be purely *freedom from . . .* the demands of others. As an individual, I have the psychocultural tendency to gather into myself power in order to define myself as an individual, to say to myself, "Here I am. This is me. I am self-made and free of any attempt by others to make me do for them what I don't want to do." I seek ego density and weight to assure my identity. I seek to avoid the weakness of weakness: decentering, uselessness, giving way, incompetence, and impotence.

As an ego, I focus my understanding solely from the point of view of my ego. Seated in the control booth of my consciousness, intentionally directing myself with my panoramic view of what is before me, I *comprehend* my world to make good judgments and right choices, and avoid those obsessively feared bad choices. My visual reach totally grasps my field of vision. I *comprehend.*

In my locus of power, I exert concentrated effort to *control* my world to achieve success, as opposed to failure. I expend energy to *control,* to make use of what I get my hands on, to feed my hungers, to manipulate both crude and sophisticated technologies.

Above all, I *consume* those goods to satisfy my needs in order to guarantee the fullest enjoyment and happiness of life, as opposed to suffering.

I *consume* by changing the nature of the goods in themselves into goods for me. The apple becomes me. The hammer becomes mine. Although driven to *comprehend, control,* and *consume,* I find I cannot exercise that much power over my world. My field of vision holds mysteries because the things in it are partially hidden behind other things, and are seen differently by other people from their own perspectives. The objects in my hands leave wastes I do not intend in the paths of other people. The ingredients of my pleasures bring unintended consequences, and the needs of others have greater rights over mine. My world is beyond my *comprehension,* my *control,* my *consumption,* because those other persons, who make the rest of the world significant, are beyond my comprehension, control and consumption. My powers are exposed as illusory.

Although *exposed,* I still feel driven to the seductive and illusory need to comprehend, control, and consume. I must *confess* that I tend, unjustifiably in the face of this *exposure* by others, and against my own best understanding, to claim all the power of my knowledge, effort, and satisfaction to my ego-centered existence; and I must *confess* this tendency.

Briefly, having been humbled by being *exposed* as tending toward ego-centered violence, what do I discover in my reflection on my experience of the call of the Other as a command? I discover that my deepest *understanding* begins from the awe of the infinite *incomprehensibility* of the Other. Wisdom begins with the mystery and dignity of the Other announcing *infinite otherness* to me in the beyond-phenomenon of her face. My greatest *success* is the sacrifice of selfishness to serve the needs of the absolutely *uncontrollable,* yet needy Other. My richest *enjoyment* is the celebration of the satisfaction of the neediest needs of the *unconsumable* Other. When I use power to achieve my own density rather than to transcend my egocentric habits, I implode and destroy my own power. When I return the power invested in me by the Other and direct it toward the good of the Other, I authentically find myself.

Discovered selfishness in ourselves shames us. The opportunity to retreat from selfishness and give to another makes us all sigh with relief from our own self-destructiveness. My students tell me they grow more in self-knowledge from their service-learning activities than from their focused self-developing study.

This argument that the *exposure* of my self-destructive striving for ego-centered power is what weakens me, this paradox of the weakness of power, needs careful unfolding with the help of Levinas's distinctions between *totality* and *infinity,* and between *need* and *desire.*

As an ego-centered self I define myself as the *subject,* the one who acts upon all that is not me as subject, that is, *objects.* I, the *subject,* know, manipulate, and enjoy those things that are other than me. I define all others (things and persons) as *objects* available to my understanding, effort, and satisfaction. Claiming my power to myself, I totalize (objectify) others. I claim others to be *nothing-more-than* what I make them to be. As an ego-centered self I try to *comprehend* (totally grasp in understanding), I try to *control* (totally dominate by my own effort), and I try to *consume* (satisfy my needs by total use of others).

I too often define myself as the *subject* and the other person as my *object*. However, when I egologically reduce my experience of her as an independent *subject* to being an object for my needs, I find myself conflicted in my effort to respond to my deepest desire. While, on the one hand, I try to reduce the Other to an *object*, simultaneously, on the other hand, I desire her to be a *subject*. I desire her to be interesting and exciting. I want her to be one who knows, chooses, acts upon, and enjoys things in life, especially with me. While I think I want to *comprehend* the other, simultaneously I desire her to create meanings independent of me. Only an independent and mysterious Other is *uncomprehendably* interesting and able to be known and desired.

While I think I want to *control* the other, simultaneously I desire her to exercise independent and creative action. Only an independently willing Other is *uncontrollably* able to act with me, rather than by me. I want her behavior to surprise me, to be unanticipated, to be purely gratuitous. Her actions must be gifts in order for me to experience gratitude, that sense of joy for receiving what I neither expected nor deserved.

Finally, while I think I want to *consume* the Other, feast off her delectable qualities to enjoy her, simultaneously I desire her to be enigmatically and creatively imaginative, escaping any of my own or others' tricks to consume her. I do not want to be satisfied and thus satiated by her. I want my desire for her to be insatiable, to deepen rather than fill my desire. Only an independent Other is *unconsumably* enjoyable.

Even this expression of wanting her to be independent can be a violation of her independence. Her *otherness*, her absolute independence is not a result of my wanting, my *desire*. She is independent. I *find* her to be an *uncomprehendable, uncontrollable*, and *unconsumable* Other. The origin of her independent otherness is in her, not in my *desire*. My *desire* is not a strong need trying to be respectful. The origin of my *desire* comes from her being *desirable*, which comes to me from her *epiphany* (*epi-* "to, unto" + *phainein* "to show"), the absolute showing forth from her to me of her independent goodness.

I get caught in the conflict between, on the one hand, what I think to be my justifiable search for need fulfillment from the Other, and, on the other hand, my transcendent *desire* for her good as other, which *desire* is a *finding* from her epiphany. My ego-centered needs, on the one hand, are my tendencies to relate to the Other as an object, to claim my power to make her be *nothing-more-than* that which can fill my lacks. My other-centered desire, on the other hand, is my possibility to find her to be an infinitely other subject. I find I receive my power from others who are *always-more-than* that which is to fill my own needs. I want to use my power to be responsible to and for others who are *always-more-than* my ego-centered needs.

But this interpretation that I am caught in a dilemma is an ego-seduction and illusion. I misinterpret that I am caught in a contradiction between two mutually exclusive tendencies: drives to fill ego-needs, and desire-for-the-other-as-Other. Power, indeed, must be used to fill needs; but the misuse of power can reduce the Other to an object. The resolution of the conflict begins as I find, not only that I do not want to *reduce* the Other to an object for my subjective self, but also that she is, by her very nature as other, *irreducible.* I recognize how I can defeat myself because, at the deepest level of my being, the Other is experienced not as an object, but as a subject, another free person whose existence is an infinite independence from my needy ego.

In the experience of power moving from the center of me to the center of the Other, the experience of my power as a subject over her as an object moving to recognize her as an independent subject, in this radical Copernican shift of axis, I myself take on the likeness of an object for the Other. When I find the helpless infant, I become objectlike, the means, the tool for her need fulfillment. The infant becomes the subject: the one needing, the one demanding, the one whose infinite dignity and yet neediness is calling me to be for her. This shift is not easy. Being reduced to an objectlike existence is experienced as suffering, and I often react defensively to preserve *myself-as-subject* in the manner I had previously deluded myself: one who relates to the Other as an object for my subjectivity.

But I discover that this is not that kind of radical shift of axis, where I am transformed into an object for another subject. That kind of transformation would preserve a totalizing structure, with only the roles being reversed. That would be the kind of pathological relationship the authors of the codependency books rage about in which the person loses her independence by serving the other. Responding to the call to care for the needs of another does not have to reduce me to an object. I find I am an authentic source of being a subject when I am of service to others. My identity is not lost; I am identified as the one called at this moment to freely serve the needs of the Other, and the one responding to these needs. My subjectivity is not turned into objectivity. It is subjectivity in its most authentic form. My freedom is not reduced; it is freed. My will is not corrupted; it is consecrated. "The other's physical needs are my spiritual needs" (an old Jewish proverb Levinas is fond of quoting).

If I am caught in the trap of the selfishness of my own ego, I reduce myself to being most like an object. When I categorically reduce others to stereotypes, I am most like the mindless machinelike calculator. When I manipulate others with my force, I am most like a bulldozer with its irresistible physical strength. When I simply feed my needs to nourish my feeding, I am most like a vegetable transforming nutrients into my cellular structure. When I am most like an object, I cannot respond to the needs of the infant. I have weakened myself.

This revelation of the paradoxical reveals the authentic *psukhe*: the breather of the spirit of others. To unpack the psukhe's ability to sabotage itself, and to redeem itself in its relations to others, we need a *psukhology* of the weakness of power and of the power of weakness.

THE WEAKNESS OF POWER

Power that claims freedom to be self-generating and self-directing weakens itself. I tend to center myself on my needs and give these needs priority over my desire for others. I reduce others to a totality (an object for myself as subject) and I miss the Other's infinity (a subject always beyond my own capricious subjectivity).

Ego-centered power is power assumed in what the phenomenologists call "the natural attitude." Caught up in the business of responding to and fulfilling my own needs, I tend to locate my center in myself. I act as if I were the hub of my world and I intend (direct myself) toward all other things and persons from that central place. I assume the basis for all my experience is my *intentionality*, my intending out from this center. All others are seen from this vantage point. All others are evaluated from this standard. All others are means to my ends as pragmatic goals of my free subjectivity. I am the doer of acts for the accomplishment of my freedom. All others are enjoyed depending on the value of their qualities to satisfy my needs as an organic and psychological consumer.

Before describing the root of the weakness of the power of this ego-centered self, I will further describe this egological tendency toward power in the three orders of the psyche, borrowing from mythology and other authors and psychologists to describe the psychological complexes.

At the level of knowing, my ego-centered *intelligence*, rather than *understanding* others, tends to be arrogant and obsessive, self-righteous in judgments of others and defensive against their calling my ego into question. This is the *Gyges complex*.

At the level of acting, my ego-centered *effort*, rather than *successful* in relationships, tends to be manipulative and compulsive, demanding results that abuse and alienate others. This is the *Zeus complex.*

At the level of feeling, my ego-centered *satisfaction* of needs, rather than bringing *happiness*, tends to be greedy and addictive, an indulgence that becomes decadent, repulsive to others, and self-destructive. This is the *Narcissus complex.*

The Gyges Complex: Self-righteous and Obsessive

Self-righteousness: my intelligence is exposed as arrogant and obsessive and I confess my tendency to reduce others.

My ego-centered righteousness is the claim that my choices are based on truth created by my own powers of knowing from the superior vantage point of my own situation. I am *certain* of my truth. I tend to claim that my meanings are not received from others. My ego-centered righteousness denies my knowledge of the world to be a gift from otherness itself (the otherness of the world and especially the otherness of my multiple teachers, all others) and, therefore, to be shared with others. My ego-centered righteousness does not recognize that knowledge is public and gratuitous, just as the world is common and free. When I am captured by ego-centered individualism I do not experience gratitude toward others for their generosity in sharing their understanding of the world, nor is there any generosity on my part in giving back that understanding to still other others. My ego-centered righteousness deceives me into believing that I know what others do not know, that my knowledge is solely the product of my own marvelous constituting intelligence. It assumes others are ignorant about what I know. Ego-centered righteousness is the *seduction* of *arrogant comprehension* that reduces others to my *certain* knowledge. This seduction of comprehension and certainty is what we might call the *Gyges complex.*

Let me briefly retell the story of the Greek myth of Gyges, from whom came the name for this habit of understanding self and others that is basically ego-centered and self-deceived. Gyges was a shepherd in service to the King of Lydia in Asia Minor. While tending his sheep following an earthquake, he came upon a cleft in the ground. He entered into a large cavern where he found a hollow bronze horse. Inside the horse lay a larger than life corpse of a man. On the man's finger, Gyges found a ring, which he took off and placed on his own finger. He returned above ground to his fellow herdsmen. As he played with the ring on his finger, he soon found it had magical power. When he turned the ring to hide the bezel in his palm, he himself became invisible! When he turned it back to the outside, he became visible again! To make this story short, Gyges, with this extraordinary power to turn himself into an *unseen seer*, left his dumb sheep, went to the capital, stole into the castle, made love to the queen, killed the impotent king, and took over the kingdom (Grant and Hazel, 1973, p. 191). What a great story to reveal to us our tendency toward arrogance.

Psychologists use the notion of a *complex* to indicate a psychological pattern in which a person narrowly interprets situations and rigidly behaves in them. This pattern locks the person into tendencies that can be identified and explained by previous events in their life, events usually traumatic. A good example is Freud's notion of the Oedipus complex, in which the male child fears his father and attaches himself to his mother.

Levinas reintroduces the ancient Greek myth of Gyges to describe the tendency of the ego to retreat to a hidden and safe interior vantage place from which to look out at and judge others. He says, "The myth of Gyges is the very myth of the I and interiority, which exist non-recognized" (1961/1969, p. 61). As a psychologist, I take this philosophical notion retrieved from mythology to define a pattern I find in myself of interpreting and behaving. I find a complex.

The *Gyges complex* is the operational belief that I can see the meanings of others, and yet keep mine hidden from their perception. I consider myself fairly observant and perceptive of the personality characteristics of others and the meanings they express about their surrounding world. Simultaneously, I consider myself fairly good at hiding my own intentions, feelings, and beliefs from the perception of others. I think I can penetrate the disguises of others, while keeping them from peering into my inner self. I am the one who sees without being seen, an *unseen seer*.

Plato used the story of Gyges to ask if we only act morally when we know others are watching and, possibly, act immorally if confident that others would not see our misdeeds. I can use the Gyges myth to ask nearly the same thing of myself: Do I not act in ways founded on the assumption that my bodily behavior may well be visible and my mental intentions invisible? Do I also not act with confidence that my piercing observations of the bodily behavior of others and my psychological intelligence can figure out the intentions of others?

I must note that psychologists recognize the opposite of the Gyges complex to be a pathological characteristic. Some people have the inordinate fear of being quite transparent, even penetrable by the eyes of others. They have lost their boundaries. This extreme boundary-less self is symptomatic of the schizoid personality.

Most of us, while finding the Gyges complex of the unseen seer to be logically self-contradictory, still act a bit like the voyeur Gyges. We pride ourselves on our ability to peer through the veiled actions of others to see their private intentions, while we remain safely behind our masks beyond their view. We consider ourselves fairly perceptive *psychologists* reading others like books, and fairly clever *actors* disguising our true selves behind a self-confident fiction.

The Gyges complex is both a *seduction* and a *delusion*. As an ego-centered self, I deceive myself about my exaggerated ability to be perceptive and simultaneously hidden. I falsely believe I can arrogantly show off my comprehensive and certain understanding of reality, and I assume others cannot see the source of my knowledge. I reason that, since others cannot see inside my head, they cannot see my dependence on others for my understanding of the world. As an ego-centered self I claim to be my own source of knowledge about the world. I claim that my knowledge is the product of my constituting consciousness and that, therefore, I can freely alter my description of the world. I think I can alter knowledge, at least in telling others, to give me an advantage. When I tell a *lie* I am assuming my knowledge is hidden from others.

But to be a successful liar, I must be an extraordinarily confident Gyges, too confident. Knowledge is not a product of my consciousness. My source of knowledge is from the world by way of other persons. The Gyges complex is the self-captured and self-deceptive belief that I can lie and not be witnessed. Ego-centered understanding mistakenly justifies my self-righteous choices. Self-righteousness justifies its own attempt to deceive others.

However, since I am not Gyges, since my intentions are far more available to perceptive others than what I self-deceptively imagine, and since the common world is certainly as available to others as to myself, then my lies are likely detected and the power I hoped to gain is sabotaged. Choices based on the self-deception that my lies are believed by others usually lash back upon my later choices. My lies catch up with me. I am *exposed* as self-deceptive and my power is shown to be weak.

I deceive myself the most when I try to act sincere. My most self-deceptive lie resides in my efforts toward sincerity. James Hatley, in a yet unpublished paper (1996), points out Levinas's concern about the insincerity of sincerity. Hatley says that "the greatest danger to one's conscience," as characterized by Levinas, "lies not in its possible insincerity but in a feigned pose of naiveté" (p. 8). Hatley further remarks that

> even more dangerous than the danger of a troubled and troubling insincerity is that sincerity that is content, that assumes its innocence, that does not acknowledge its own vulnerability to insincerity. Indeed, this sort of sincerity is the very gesture of insincerity. Thus, what one normally terms insincerity, i.e. a

deception that covers over one's intentions in relation to the other, begins not simply with a deception of the other but of oneself as well. (p. 9)

The Zeus Complex: Manipulative and Compulsive

Manipulative: my effort is exposed as self-driven and compulsive and I confess my tendency for violence.

My ego-centered demands claim that my successes are the result of my abilities exclusively developed by my own exertion of effort. I do not readily admit that my successes are created out of the conditions set by others, and I do not credit others when I use my abilities exclusively for my own ends. I resist the experience of gratitude to others for helping me develop my successful capabilities and resist any generosity with those abilities. My ego-centered effort comes from believing I am a *self-made man*. I do not allow myself to admit my dependence on others, not only for my knowledge, but also for my native intelligence and skills and my developed habits. I tend to act with too much belief in self-creation and self-importance. I am seduced by my successes. I convince myself that these successes are the outcome of my intelligent knowing and willful action, and therefore are my right to exclusive enjoyment. This seduction is grounded on the belief that my individual freedom is the essential characteristic of my existence. I convince myself that my freedom takes priority over every other value. Even when I try to be responsible, I claim my responsibility is the product of my free choice. I am in control of my life. My ego-centered demanding is the *seduction* of manipulative *control.* This style of self-conviction about godlike freedom, this belief of being totally in charge, this *seduction toward compulsive control* is called the *Zeus complex.*

My Zeus complex is my belief that my successful capabilities give me special rights that exempt me from the strict adherence to rules expected of others in an ordered community. I am privileged, special, and precious. My Zeus complex does not urge me to think I am more powerful in the sense of physical might. But it does urge me to think I am able to place myself above the law, above the mores and morals of my society. These regulations hold for ordinary people in ordinary circumstance. Indeed, I abide by them in ordinary circumstances when other people see me as ordinary. But given my ability to recognize my special circumstances, in the privileged place of my Gyges-like consciousness, I sometimes justify exemptions of some rules. I set them aside. If nobody is looking, why not? My arrogant and manipulative ego takes others as means to my ends, and I claim success. My ego-centered arrogance justifies my abuse of others to successfully serve my own needs. It justifies my demanding to do what I want.

Zeus was the Greek god who, although not strictly the father of the other gods, since he had brother and sister and cousin gods, nor even the creator of humankind, still set himself up as the supreme ruler. He punished other gods and pretty much dealt with humans by a capricious will rather than by the rules set for the maintenance of order. Although he was fairly benevolent and impartial, still he considered himself above the law (Grant and Hazel, 1973, pp. 418–23).

We all engage in a little Zeus-complex activity. We expect others to stick to the rules governing fairness, but exempt our special selves if we see a clear advantage, especially if we can get away with not being seen by others, or are able to rationalize our privileged grounds for exemption. We reject authority over ourselves. We tend to honor our freedom above any obedience and resist calculations of equality with others. Although we assume an implicit contract of reciprocity with other, since we cannot know how to exactly divide reciprocal responsibility and benefit, we tend to make sure we neither do too much nor get too little.

Certainly, there are those who seem pathologically unable to rule even the smallest corners of their own lives and are totally manipulatable by others. The catatonic is malleable, fearful of the potential harm of his own actions, unresistant to orders from others.

Although I may recognize this Zeus complex of claiming some special status to be irrational, I still act in ways that set me apart from others. I reserve for myself, at least in my own consciousness, a privileged status. I act as if I were Number One, in spite of evidence that places me lesser than others.

The Zeus complex is both a *seduction* and a *delusion*. As an ego-centered self, I deceive myself about my exaggerated ability to be decisive and determined in my effort for success. I falsely believe my freedom originates in my ego. The origin of my freedom is not in myself. It is invested in me by the needs of others. I am not like Zeus. And, since I am not really like Zeus, exempt from the social rules of behavior while holding others to them, my behavior as someone special makes me isolated and lonely. My ego-centered demanding alienates others and is self-isolating. I am *exposed* as self-defeating, and my power has become weakness.

The Narcissus Complex: Self-indulgent and Addictive

Self-indulgent: my satisfaction is exposed as greedy and addictive and I confess my tendency to be selfish.

My ego-centered indulging claims that my satisfaction is the well
deserved reward of my own choices and the success of my own effort. I
claim that the good things that happen to me do not come from others, nor
do I feel obliged to offer them for the satisfaction of others. As an ego-
centered self, I claim the right to privately enjoy my satisfaction. I do not
experience gratitude for, or generosity with, my own satisfaction. Ego-
centered indulging is the *seduction* of *greedy consumption*. This greediness
is called the *Narcissus complex*.

My *Narcissus complex* is my excessive admiration of myself. My satisfied sensuousness is all that is needed for my enjoyment. I get totally
absorbed by my own self-satisfaction. My addictions consume me as they
consume what they enjoy.

Narcissism is well known to clinicians as a common pathology that is
difficult to treat. Freud resurrected the Greek myth of Narcissus to name
his understanding of self-love. Narcissus was the beautiful lad who,
though courted by many, repulsed them all, and contemplated his own
beauty reflected in a pool on Mount Helicon. The more he looked, the
deeper he fell in love with himself. This futile passion held him in its grip,
as he lay day after day on a rock beside the pool, until he wasted away and
died (Grant and Hazel, 1973, p. 285).

Certainly there are those who seem the opposite of Narcissus, pathologically unable to enjoy themselves at all. They are filled with guilt after
satisfying any need. Neurotic guilt can make self-denial an ego-centered
style.

The Narcissus complex is both a *seduction* and a *delusion*. As an ego-
centered self, I am deceived by my exaggerated ability to enjoy myself
through the exclusive satisfaction of my own needs. In reality, authentic
enjoyment is experienced only in celebrating with others the satisfaction
of their needs. Paradoxically, isolated enjoyment feeds off others who are
seen as convenient commodities or at least service providers of goods for
my enjoyment. The self-indulgence of exclusive self-satisfaction reduces
others to objects supporting freedom to enjoy. This self-indulgence is self-
destructive, because it consumes that which is the source of enjoyment by
the self: the freely enjoying other. When I am greedy, I am *exposed* and my
power becomes weak.

HOW POWER WEAKENS POWER

My ego-centered power is weak because I fail to see that authentic power
is received from others, and because I do not reinvest this gratuitously
given power in others for their understanding, success, and enjoyment.

When I fail to experience gratitude (the power of acknowledging my gra-tuitously received power), and generosity (the power of graciously giving back power), I deny relationship, the only condition in which power is authentically powerful. Ego-centered power, fulfilling only the needs of my ego and rejecting relationship with others, weakens the five general ways I increase my freedom in these interpersonal relationships. I sabo-tage my own individual power. The power of individual knowledge, action, and feeling is paradoxically weak. This weakness is found in (1) *self-absorbed centering,* (2) *ego-serving service,* (3) *ego-demanding reciprocity,* (4) *ego-driven winning,* and, (5) *ego-dominated authority.*

Self-Centering Becomes Ego-Absorbed

When I become so captured in my efforts for self-improvement, intending to serve exclusively my own needs, then I isolate myself further from rela-tionship with others and lose my source of power. Knowledge and skills have their source in others and are to be used to bind myself to others in relationships of mutual interdependence. Knowledge originating from attending to the needs of others has a priority over knowledge from atten-tion to my own needs. This priority of the Other over the self does not describe a physical hierarchy. Nor does it necessarily mean a temporal priority. It does mean an ethical priority.

For knowledge to be *objective,* it must be detached from ego-interest. Ego-interested knowledge is always vulnerable to distortion by my narrow needs. Ego-directed activity is vulnerable to stubborn drive for success. Ego-nourishing satisfaction is vulnerable to self-corroding indulgence. Self-improvement must be a means to serve others; it is not an end in itself. When self-improvement becomes its own goal, it is self-destructive.

Nor should my self-improvement become a means exclusively for more self-improvement. I can become driven toward those small incre-ments of gain in the midst of self-improving activities and lose sight of the ultimate value of an improved ability. There is often a vicious cycle in my self-improvement. This is the paradoxical weakness of the power of *cen-tering.* When I focus my attention toward myself to improve my own abil-ities solely for ego-improvement and not for serving the needs of others, my obsessive tendency toward constant improvement destroys itself. My attention gets focused on the satisfactions of little steps of improvement, while I become inexhaustively needy for more success in improvement. Self-improvement can get addictive.

EGO-OBSESSION

When, at the level of knowing, my self-reflecting becomes ego-centered centering, it isolates, absorbs, and weakens me. When I disregard the meanings of others, which, at the most fundamental level, provide an understanding of their reality, then I superimpose meaning on them to fit my needs. Ego-centered centering self-righteously reduces others to stereotypes and replaces their meanings with the fictions that support the ego's interests. This kind of centering deceives itself about reality.

In actuality, I have no independent access for understanding reality. I know it only by way of others. My perceptual and rational processes are not opened toward the world by the individual force of my isolated and needy will. They are unlocked from the Other and I am invited out by the Other calling me to respond to her needs. The door to knowledge has the knocker only on the outside. The origin of my intention to see and hear comes from the other person drawing my senses out to those things as objects capable of fulfilling her needs.

My obsessively ego-centered ego, Gyges-like, the one that depends on my own source of power to direct my perceptual attention, sees and hears a distorted reality. My neediness warps my perceptions and ideas. Ego-centered understanding gets narrow-minded and captured inside its own knowledge. There is nothing more self-deceptive than self-righteous understanding.

EGO-COMPULSION

When, at the level of acting, my self-directing becomes ego-centered centering, it isolates, absorbs, and weakens me, because I deny the needs of others, which are, at the most fundamental level, the authentic motivators of effort. In reality, I have no motivation to act independent of others, but am drawn out (moved) by the desire to serve others. Ultimately, without others, I have no reason to live. Behavior is not the individual force of an isolated and needy will. It is not driven from within, but drawn from without to respond to the call of the needful Other.

My compulsively centered ego, Zeus-like, the one caught in my own source of power, cannot break my ritual patterns. Actions found to be successful on their own terms and taken as self-originating get routinized and driven. Well-developed habits offer the ease of less effort, but they can deceive me into a complacency of successful, repetitious action. The needs of others, which call for alternative actions, go unattended because I am caught up in my own success. There is nothing more potentially deceptive than a successful style of self-improving action.

EGO-ADDICTION

When, at the level of feeling, my self-nourishing becomes ego-centered centering, narcissistically captured, it isolates, absorbs and weakens me, because it loses the reality that the fulfillment of the needs of others, at the most fundamental level, is the occasion for celebration. Alone, I cannot satisfy myself enough to provide for my enjoyment. Enjoyment is the most fundamental ingredient of gratitude. It is the pure experience of gratuitousness; that which is enjoyed offers a pure gift. It is no product of my doing. The pleasurable comes from somewhere beyond me; it gives its gift to me. My receiving it as a gift, as a purely given benefit, is grateful enjoyment. Gratitude seeks expression. I desire to celebrate satisfaction with others. The voraciously centered ego gets only a temporary and shallow satisfaction and cannot truly enjoy itself. Since *desire*, the intention to fulfill others' needs, has ethical priority over the intention to fulfill my own needs, my ego-centered satisfaction represses my desire for the fulfillment of the needs of others.

My addictively centered self, Narcissus-like, the one that indulges in satisfying only my own pleasure (satiation), becomes insatiable, dulled, and complacent. There is nothing more self-deceptive than my fully satisfied self. When satisfied, I get fat and happy, but it is a happiness that corrodes my deepest human characteristic, my desire for the good of others. Ego-centered nourishing is addiction.

Serving Others Becomes Ego-Serving

When the goal of my serving becomes the fulfillment of my own need to define myself as a generous server, I miss the needs of the served and sabotage my service. As authentic server I must attend to my service, but always for the purpose of fulfilling the needs of the served. My service, coming from my own need to be a server, is weak because I tend to serve what I, as server, want to serve, but not necessarily what the one served needs. In the worst case, I get captured in this project of self definition. I serve badly, and then, when the one served complains, I judge her to be unreceptive and ungrateful for my service.

As a server of others, I am caught in the tension between attending to the proper goal of my service, the fulfillment of the other's needs, and attending to my own activity in striving to provide my best service. The needs and satisfaction of the Other cannot be fully known, yet I seek them in order to serve. Others are *always-more-than* what I can know and serve. This is the paradox of the powerlessness of serving. When others are reduced to *nothing-more-than* the occasion for me to define myself as a server, I am paradoxically weakened. I am *exposed* as a self-serving server, and sabotage my service.

EGO-SERVING INSTRUCTION

When, at the level of knowing, my teaching of another becomes ego-centered serving, it descends into irrelevancy, because I disregard the other's need for meaning, which originally drew forth my teaching. In ego-centered instruction, I define myself as the one who knows the needs of the Other, and instruct her according to this definition, rather than according to her needs, whose meanings are revealed to me by her. I can sabotage my service and weaken myself as an instructor when I assume that I understand the needs of the Other and that I, from my arrogant position as *expert*, know her meanings better than she knows her own meanings. When my understanding originates from my need to be an expert and teacher, without being guided by the needs of the Other, then the knowledge I tell her has no value for her. Ego-serving instruction fails to serve because the Other cannot be an object to receive the action of my ego-centered power.

When I do not understand the Other, I blame her as the cause of my ignorance, claiming that she has not expressed her needs. Since her expressions do not fit my prior self-generated knowledge of her, I conclude she is resisting my teaching. My ignorance comes from my arrogantly sophisticated interpretation. But I blame her. Her attempts to express her own meanings are further interpreted as resistance. This often provokes me, and, as *expert*, I try harder to convince her. The more I try to instruct her, the less I understand and the less I am able to adequately instruct. My lessons are irrelevant, and therefore I weaken myself as a server. The word *propoganda* comes from *pro-* ("forth") + *pangere* ("to fasten"). My propaganda, my instruction to fasten onto others what I think they need, based on the advantage to me as instructor, is self-weakening power.

EGO-SERVING HELPING

When, at the level of acting, my helping becomes ego-centered serving, it can harm, or at least, hinder the Other, because I disregard her needs, which are, at the most fundamental level, the original and authentic motivators of my helping. In ego-centered, skillful helping, I define myself as the one whose skills are most proper for the Other's success, rather than aiding the skills of the Other, whose abilities are proper for her success. I can sabotage my serving and weaken myself as a helper when I exert effort with those skills that succeed in expressing my clever ability but are not guided by the needs of the Other. My ego-centered use of abilities cannot change the Other's needs to fit these abilities. When my skills originate from my need to be a helper without being guided by the Other's needs, then the help I offer cannot adequately serve. Ego-serving skills fail to serve the Other, because the Other cannot be an object for the action of my ego-centered power.

This failure to serve the Other is often interpreted by me as due to the resistance of the other to receive help, and I, as an ego-centered *helper*, try harder. The more I try to help her, the less I succeed in providing for her needs. Her increased neediness, affected by my persistence in forcing my skills on her, entices me as a potential place to exercise my generous help. I often try even harder to manipulate her behavior to benefit my needs. The harder I try to control the other with my own ego-directed skills, the less I am able to change her. My ego-centered skills are improper for the helped, and therefore they weaken me as helper.

EGO-SERVING PROVIDING

When, at the level of feeling, my giving to another becomes ego-centered providing, my giving gives inappropriate gifts, because I disregard her needs, which are, at the most fundamental level, the original and authentic inspiration of my providing. In ego-centered giving, I define myself as the one whose feelings are to enjoy, rather than to compassionately provide for the enjoyment of the Other. I can sabotage my giving and weaken myself as a giver when I give ego-centered gifts, because I attempt to satisfy my need to be a generous giver. But when these gifts are not appropriate to the needs of the receiver, I weaken my satisfaction as a generous giver. The satisfaction of giving is found in fulfilling the receiver's needs. Ego-centered giving, centered on my satisfaction as a giver rather than on the needs of the receiver, cannot bring real satisfaction to me as the giver.

The Other has independent needs, her own taste, her own kind of satisfaction. When I try unsuccessfully to force the enjoyment of what I give, I often interpret this failure of the receiver to enjoy my gifts as resistance, and I try even harder to get her to enjoy them. The independent joy of the Other arouses me, sometimes to envy and jealousy, and I try harder to enter into her joy by giving my inappropriate gifts. The harder I try to satisfy my giving, rather than celebrate the fulfillment of her needs, the less I am able to enjoy her and even my own satisfaction. Ego-centered gifts, inappropriate for the receiver, weaken the giver.

Cooperation Becomes Demanding Reciprocity

Cooperation is based more on trust than on the demand for the Other to give back to me. It is founded on the truss or support of concern for the Other, rather than on a kind of barter to assure my benefit. However, when I keep my attention primarily on demanding equal reciprocity for my receiving, and on my own giving as that which only purchases receiving, then I sabotage the cooperative venture and weaken myself. In ego-centered *cooperation*, I try to exercise my power for the Other to expend more, or at least equal, sacrifice, and for myself to receive more, or at least equal, benefit. This behavior is arrogant, manipulative, and greedy.

In true cooperation, each partner knows that success is not possible alone. The success of cooperation rests on each attending to giving to the Other and trusting that the Other will share. The tension of cooperation is in contributing without demanding reciprocity, yet enjoying the success that could only be gained with the Other's contribution. When I center my attention on receiving, because I believe my greatest need is to use the benefits of the partner with the least sacrifice from myself, then I sabotage the delicate bond of cooperation. I reject the infinite value of the Other.

Excessive attention to my cost and benefit reduces my partner to an object, to another tool to get my work done and another means to gain my own ends. Ego-centered cooperation, in which I am vying for my individual advantage can turn into vicious competition against the partner. This competition brings the loss of mutual advantage. Paradoxically, my partner exercises her *subjectivity*, gaining as much or more benefit than myself. I often find that my demanding reciprocity has induced her to play the competitive game in return, reducing me to an object for her. I am *exposed* as egoistic and am emptied of the power of cooperation.

DIALOGUE BECOMES BICKERING AND ACCUSING

At the level of knowing, my cooperation can become an ego-centered *dialogue*, where I, as speaker, am more intent upon defending my position, persuading the other for the sake of self-gain, than on seeking the truth. Real dialogue is cooperative discussion for mutual understanding of the actual state of affairs, the truth of reality. But when I am captured by my need to protect my power, I can turn the discussion into competition to win some point over the Other. Ego-centered dialogue is weak because it does not gain any mutually clear understanding. It turns out to be, at worst, a double monologue: two people speaking, each listening only to her/himself, but not to each other.

A dialogue, where one is a self-centered participant and the Other is centered on seeking the truth, frustrates the honest one and self-sabotages the egoist. When my motive to persuade supersedes my motive to seek the truth, my ego-centered speaking is founded on the assumption that I am *certain* that this person is blindly gullible, that she does not grasp my egological intention to convince rather than reveal truth. This is a self-weakening assumption. Another can likely see through this rhetoric. I am *exposed* as egoistic.

My lies expose my Gyges complex: my foolish belief that my intentions are invisible while I envision the psyche of the Other. This belief is risky. Some rhetoricians are clever and convince the gullible. But gullibility itself is foolish. The listener's gullibility is founded on her greater need to be willing to accept whatever is said than to seek the truth. The rhetorician convinces only the foolish but is a fool to the insightful. There is no weaker position than to feign cooperation in discussion, to appeal to the trust of the listener and then to violate that trust with dishonesty. The authentic listener will likely penetrate all this deceit and be convinced the speaker is a liar. Caught in deceptive rhetoric, the self loses credibility and is greatly weakened.

COLLABORATING BECOMES MANEUVERING AND GETTING REVENGE

At the level of acting, ego-centered *collaboration*, which has turned into jockeying for position to assure reciprocity for ego-gain, weakens the self. Real collaboration is cooperation of labor founded on trust to gain a common goal. My ego-centered maneuvering undercuts mutual trust, sabotages the joint project, and weakens me. When I am captured by my need to empower myself, I turn the action into competition to get my partner to contribute more than what I give. In maneuvering, I intend to succeed while using the Other to be a means (object) for my success, and simultaneously ensuring that I am not used as a means for the success of the Other. My demand for her reciprocity forces the Other to demand my reciprocity. In this maneuvering for individual advantage, we abandon the trust necessary for cooperation.

My ego-centered manipulation *exposes* my Zeus complex: demanding trust from the Other while exempting myself from the same interpersonal rule of good conduct. But, first of all, paradoxically, I often discover myself outmaneuvered. I discover my assumed position of being special and above the rules of cooperation to be itself reduced from being special by the Other: I find myself manipulated and weak. From this condition of sabotaged maneuvering, I seek revenge. My demand for reciprocity from my partner who has turned my ego-centered maneuvering to her advantage arouses my vengeance, and I try even more deceitful maneuvers to get even. Or I find the Other seeing through my manipulative efforts and abandoning me. I am left without a partner for collaboration. The seduction and illusion of control of the Other in what ought to be a cooperative venture ultimately defeats me.

The greatest self-deceptive paradox occurs when, in a successful ploy of maneuvering, I find my victim correlatively motivated to turn coopera- tion into an inverted competition: while I deceptively seek to win, she deceptively seeks to lose. She seeks to be a *willing victim*. Beating a willing victim, in a project originally calling for cooperation, sabotages even an opportunity for revenge. The willing victim paradoxically wins. The vic- tor, whose victory is willed by the victim, loses. Family fighting built on long histories of competition rather than on cooperation, in which the roles of losers and winners have been long practiced, turning into vicious codependency supporting the sham roles of victims and victors, are deeply self-destructive.

DIVIDING GOODS BECOMES GRASPING AND STINGY

At the level of feeling, my *cooperative* division of goods can become an ego- centered effort to get more than the partner. This ego-centered sharing turns into cheating to divide the goods to guarantee my individual satis- faction. Real sharing is celebrating, enjoying by prizing and consuming together the goods of success. Mutual satisfaction can be the basis for mutual enjoyment, the authentic expression of gratitude for the gift of the common reward, celebration of happiness. The word *celebrate* comes from the Latin *celebrare* "to frequent, to fill together frequently." But when I am driven by my demand to fulfill my needs without regard for the Other, I turn my sharing into grasping in order to get more of the goods than the Other.

This egoistic enjoyment at the expense of the Other *exposes* my Narcissus complex: I am in love with myself and denying the Other. Ego- centered sharing is self-indulgent. But turning sharing into grasping is risky. On the one hand, I can discover the Other to be quicker at satisfying herself at my expense. On the other hand, when I consume the Other's share, I can find my victim to be taking advantage of me by fulfilling her need to be submissive. This paradoxically robs me of the opportunity to be greedy. Greed is made not only of acquisition but also of envy of the Other's goods. When the Other relinquishes her share, I may get the goods, but I am denied the desire for cooperation. Enjoying alone turns out to be worse than empty; it is self-destructive.

Competition Becomes Driven to Win

Competitors compete to win, but within the conditions that maintain the competition. When my need to win gets greater than the advantage of our mutual challenge for the sake of our mutual benefit and the common good, I weaken myself. Real competition rests on implicit or explicit rules to maintain fairness to keep the contest alive in order to serve the Other with a challenge. But when my competition turns into an effort to really beat, to oppress the Other, without regard for the rules that maintain the Other's opportunity to compete, then I lose the Other's challenge and weaken myself. First, I take the risk of being weakened in defeat by a more powerful competitor. Second, since my motive is solely to win but not at all to be challenged for the greater good of both, then, when I do win, I gain only a win. I have lost the only lasting gain from competition, the challenge to each competitor for the common good.

DEBATING BECOMES DECEIVING AND BLAMING

At the cognitive level of knowing, my debating can become an ego-centered righteousness to hide the truth from the competitor in order to win at all costs. Honest arguments are mutual challenges of ideas for greater understanding of the truth. When I strive to win by any means, rather than to seek the truth, I intend to destroy the Other's challenge of my knowledge and, paradoxically, the greater possibility to get the truth.

The seduction and illusion of so prizing a win over truth, as to lie, is self-deceptive. The deceiver assumes a lie has at least an equal, and likely a better chance than does the truth of convincing the Other. But the deceiver is more vulnerable to failure than if she admits the truth. The truth obviously has reality on its side. When the Other depends on the truth from the real world, and I depend on my lies, I not only lose the competition, but I also lose my role as an observer of the real world and as an honest debater in the search for real truth. I am *exposed* as more centered in my ego than in the world of reality. Lying, grounded on the very shaky and self-righteous Gyges complex of being an unseen seer, is especially vulnerable to self-sabotage. My recourse to lie about the origin of the falsehood, blaming it on the Other rather than myself, invites my victim to turn my double deception into a double defeat.

CONTESTING BECOMES BEATING AND HUMILITATING

At the behavioral level of acting, my contesting can become an ego-centered effort to reduce the competitor to incompetence for any challenge of my superior skill. Contests are to challenge the Other to challenge me in return for the improvement of the skills of both. When I seek to *win by any means*, when my drive to succeed annihilates the desire to compete, I intend to destroy the Other's challenge of my skills, and the greater possibility to engage in the struggle for common growth and the common good of other Others. In my effort to beat my challenger into humiliation, I not only attempt to act outside the accepted agreements to maintain the struggle, but I also intend to reduce the Other from being a subject, one with inherent dignity. Beating gains only a win and risks the loss of others as fellow strugglers against the difficulties of life for the well-being of all. Beating the Other, which is grounded on the very shaky Zeus complex, is weak. Nobody likes someone who runs up the score, or pounds the other contestant into submission. This loss of relationship weakens more than winning strengthens. Beating the Other into humiliation *exposes* me as egotistic and outside the fundamental human condition, interpersonal ethical relationship.

MARKETING/SHOPPING BECOMES HOARDING AND FLAUNTING

At the affective level of feeling satisfaction, my seeking good quality and great quantity in consuming can become an ego-centered indulging at the expense of the competitor and turn the satisfaction of needs into isolation. Consuming founded on mutual satisfaction can be a kind of mutual challenge to each other's enjoyment. Each contestant is mutually intent upon helping the Other enjoy more than they would without the challenge. But when I seek to be the only one to be satisfied, then I break the bonds of relationship. When I outconsume others by hoarding, by competitively depriving others of goods that are fundamentally common, then I gain only the opportunity to flaunt the satisfaction of narrow needs. I do not gain relationship. I thereby lose the greater possibility for genuine enjoyment: the mutual celebration of our common goods. Hoarding and flaunting *expose* my Narcissus complex and destroy my access to enjoyment with other.

Exercising Authority Becomes Authoritatively Dominating

When my egocentric use of the power of my position of authority dominates the success of the productivity and morale of my subordinates, I weaken myself as an authority. When I misuse the power invested in me by my subordinates and thereby abuse them, I sabotage my very source of power. The authentic leader is a servant. My authority gets its power only by being invested in me by those needing responsible service. Authority comes from the Latin word *augere*, meaning "to create or increase." My authority has power, but only to be used to create and increase the well-being of those over whom I exercise that power of authority and of the recipients of our corporate production. When I use that power to increase my own power at the expense of either or both groups who have invested it in me, then I no longer am a leader; I am an oppressive dictator. Oppressive power is not authority; servant leadership is authentic authority.

When, as an oppressive administrator, I find others willing to be abused, I find the weakness of those subordinates collaborating with me in sabotaging the good of the organization. This system is a *sycophantocracy*. It is too common, and it is a self-sabotaging system. When I cannot trust the subordinates to provide me with honest descriptions of the problems and successes of the organization, I lose contact with the real goal of our organization. When I cannot depend on the workers to strive for productivity, but only for good evaluations from me as the authority, I lose the opportunity for success. When I cannot share in the benefits with my subordinates because they are resentful, I lose a happy workforce. Their resentfulness feeds their sycophancy. Their sycophancy disallows them from sharing enjoyment with me, the resented authority. Their sycophancy empties my authority of any real power. The word *sycophant* names "a parasite of power who is servile and flattering of authority." It comes from the Greek *sykon* ("fig") + *phainein* ("to show"). The sycophant hides the truth behind a fig leaf while flattering the authority. When my authority inspires sycophancy, I have no followers, only resentful manipulators of my power for their own selfish gain.

When I use others as a means for my ego-centered success, then I cut myself off from relationship. Lacking relationship, in my individual power, I do not act *with* members of the organization. Acting *on* others, as if I did not belong to that community, I defeat myself. My lies become transparent, my abuse becomes rejected, and my self-indulgence becomes self-abusive and resented by others. When I try to totalize others, I am *exposed*; I am *totalized* as a *totalizer*.

EVALUATING AND PLANNING BECOMES CRITICIZING AND DECEIVING

When, as boss, I become a self-righteous *expert*, I both distrust the information my subordinates have for me, and I distrust them in using the information I should give them. My egoism reduces them to valuable partners and critically evaluate them as unworthy. I withhold, and even falsify, what they have a right to know. This deception undermines the power of my position of authority to evaluate and plan. Leadership is authentic only when the authority serves the personnel and customers by revealing information, plans, and decisions, so that the subordinates can participate in the process of guiding the activity of the organization. Negating subordinates' knowledge and withholding from them my knowledge undermines leadership.

Deception is foolish to the enlightened and convinces only the foolish. When I, Gyges-like, use my position of authority to lie (violate the investment of the freedom of truth), I isolate myself from the organization's relationships, which are held together by the investment of trust. Being outside the relationship of truth, my lie becomes transparent. I am *exposed* and am no longer the authority, even though I may have the power of the office. When I have been found out, my Gyges complex has deceived only myself. As a deceiving ego, I cannot know myself, while others know me as a deceiver and therefore have power over me. When I lie in the role of authority, I have lost my power.

MANAGING BECOMES MISHANDLING AND ABUSING

At the level of acting, my managing of materials and personnel can become an ego-centered effort for personal rather than organizational success. This mishandling and abusing breaks the trust of subordinates and customers. It corrupts the power of the authority by abusing others.

Abuse is ineffectual against the dedicated and courageous, because the courageous, motivated by the good of the organization, turn away from or defend themselves against the abuser. Abuse threatens only the cowardly. When, Zeus-like, I use my position of authority to abuse those subordinate to me, I reduce their ability to be successful. But their ability has been given over to me as the authority to serve the good of the organization and the individual members. Therefore, abusing their ability given to me denies me the very power I need to succeed. I define myself out of the accumulated power of an orderly group. When I, as an abusive authority, am no longer engaged in relational behavior that is mutually supportive, I am unable to succeed.

DISTRIBUTING BENEFITS BECOMES DEPRIVING AND CONFISCATING

At the level of feeling, my holding back benefits from the mutually contributing producers can especially abuse their rights to the profits of work. The person in authority has special access to the benefits of the organization, and therefore has ease in confiscating them.

Stealing by those in authority is greedy and repulsive to those who are generous and joyful. An authority's confiscation seduces only those who themselves are greedy. When, Narcissus-like, I use my position of authority to be greedy, I refuse to disperse back to the subordinates the rewards of organizational success. I violate the call to generosity made to me as an authority. I thereby deny myself the only possibility of enjoyment, which is the celebration of relationship, the common shared gratitude (communion). When my greed keeps me from celebrating and sharing in subordinates' shared gratitude, then others enjoy without me, and I find my Narcissus complex consumes only myself. I cannot authentically satisfy myself with goods confiscated from others, I can only indulge myself and become more isolated.

CONCLUSION

So this is the weakness of power. The method to reveal it is *confessional phenomenology*. The confessions are inspired by the goodness of the other *questioning* and *exposing* my egoism. When I recognize my tendency to place my ego-needs above the goodness of the other, then I am on the way to repairing my tendency to sabotage my own best interest.

However, *confessional phenomenology*, if taken as an end in itself, rather than as a means to prepare for service, can be itself self-serving. I can wallow in my own self-righteous understanding. I can manipulate others and myself by inspiring pity for my victimization even if it is self-victimization. I can satisfy a perverted need to enjoy the suffering of self abuse. Without service, confession of selfishness is empty.

CHAPTER SIX

The Power of Weakness

I confess my tendency to violate the rights of others.

"You do not deserve my cruelty. I took advantage of you. I'm sorry. How can I make up for the pain I caused? What can I do to help?"

It is difficult to admit selfishness. But when I am faced with the suffering of those I have hurt, they *expose* my guilt and I regret my ego-centered behavior. I have lost my temper with my children and yelled words that then embarrassed me. I have taken advantage of my generous wife, unjustly asking of her family tasks I should have done myself. My ego has gotten in the way of fairly treating students, colleagues, and administrators. I've turned my back on many who needed help. I am ashamed.

The face of the Other confronts my ego-centered tendency to violate her rights to assure my own. My freedom is *exposed* as the weakness to deceive, abuse, and indulge myself. Faced by the Other, *exposed*, I am shaken. I admit that I have not only done wrong, but that I have a tendency to do wrong. I *confess* my injury and my vices, my habits of harm.

But the face of the Other has not only *exposed* my guilt and allowed me to unburden myself with a *confession*, but also appeals to me to go beyond my guilt, to get outside of my own wretchedness, to stop feeling sorry for my selfish self, and to do something for and with her. Egologically I am traumatized. Psukhologically I am *inspired*. The face of the Other has *breathed* into me, and relieved me of my obsession to deceive, my compulsion to abuse, and my addiction to self-indulge. The face of the Other does more. She *breathes* into me a responsibility to do whatever I can, to regain my freedom, that freedom invested by and for her, to serve her and others with authenticity.

The paradox of power and weakness takes another turn: rather than banishing me because of my egocentric violence, rather than demanding that I crawl back into my hole and cover my head with the sackcloth of shame for my sins, the face of the Other calls me out of my concern for self, back to responsibility. My freedom is returned to me. I am given the opportunity to *understand* the first word of *truth* in its fullness spoken by the infinite nobility of the Other, "Do not violate me; serve me." I am given the opportunity to *exert effort* in the first movement toward *right behavior*, to serve her deserved needs. I am given the opportunity to *enjoy* the first *goodness*, the splendor of her beauty and dignity as a human person, and to celebrate together.

Contemporary psychologists urge people not to feel *guilt*; it is considered a four-letter word in the psychobabble of psychologese. If guilt remains self-focused and is the final conclusion of the confrontation by the Other whom I have hurt, then indeed, guilt is destructive. But if the face of the Other makes me feel guilty, and further inspires me out of that guilt into clearer understanding, energized effort, and celebration of her enjoyment, then guilt is essential for healing the self and authentically relating to the Other.

The vulnerability of the Other, of which I took advantage, now inspires my responsibility to relate to her worthiness and need. My interest in her is *disinterested*, without self-concern, especially without concern about what I am feeling and getting out of my interest in the Other. At the cognitive level, my search for this first word of truth is disinterested: not obsessed by my own self-interested needs. At the behavioral level, my effort toward her success is disinterested: not compulsive about my own self-interested projects. At the affective level, my enjoyment of her enjoying the fulfillment of her needs is disinterested: not addicted to my self-interested indulging of her qualities.

PHENOMENOLOGICAL METHOD: LISTENING TO, BEING TOUCHED, AND RESPONDING

What should be the phenomenological method for revealing and describing the power of her weakness to inspire me to responsibly and thus authentically relate to her? The phenomenological method of reflection revealing her reality as it exists and my relationship to her reality is *to listen to* and *be touched by* her call to be responsible. How else could I come to understand her? Having her reveal to me her dignity and needs by listening and being touched, the method to describe this reality is to *responsibly answer* her, "Here I am." Levinas refers to Isaiah 6:8 and to Samuel 1:3 for the response: *Hineni*, "Here I am." Isaiah, Samuel, and each of us respond to the call of the Other by listening, being touched, and answering. "Here I am!" means "Send me" (1974/81, p. 193n11). This is a *phenomenology of responsibility*.

The thesis of this chapter is that *the weakness of the weak is paradoxically powerful in calling me to be responsible.* Indeed, everyone knows the weakness of others, and thus it was easy, in chapter 4, to *expose* and *accuse* the weak of her weakness. In chapter 5, finding myself *exposed* as egocentric by the weakness of the Other, it was difficult, but commanded of me, to admit my weakness and *confess* my tendency toward violence. Now in chapter 6, I must reveal that which is beyond belief, the para-dox, that the very weakness of the weak is the power of the weak to inspire responsibility in me.

The child and the ill person calling me to their aid, those suffering poverty inspiring my compassion, even the irresponsibility of an enemy urging me to help them become responsible points to this paradox. Yet I only ambiguously understand these paradoxical events. I am puzzled by them. I can only point to them by *listening and being touched.* The obviousness of power and weakness in the flagrancy of the power of powerful and the suffering of the weakness of the weak nearly hides the illogical and irrational paradoxical power of weakness. Vanier's use of the notion of "the secret that the strong need the weak" is ironic. We ordinarily understand a *secret* to be some truth we know, but keep hidden from another. The *secret* of the power of the powerless is something we all know but try to keep hidden. The irony is that we hide from ourselves the fact that we egoistically fear weakness, while in actuality, weakness provides the foundation for our greatest source of power: the weakness of weak Others inspires authentic power when we serve them. I am given my true identity by the Other.

This power of weakness is not a transformation of the weakness of the weak into another kind of physical power, such that they are no longer weak but have become powerful. It is not an ontological change in them from the essence of weakness into the essence of power. It is a psukhological *conversion*, a change in our relationship. Their weakness is the same event, but turns me in a different direction. It becomes a paradox. The weakness of the Other, as weakness, is powerful. Her weakness calls me to be ethically responsible and attend to her needs.

This call is a *metaphysical command*: it is meta- (*meta-* "beyond" + *physical* "the force of nature"). It is not an *ontological demand*; it is not a power of *being* that *forces* me to respond, as an Aristotelian *efficient cause*. The call of the Other exercises *ethical* power over me. The weakness of the weak does not merely make a suggestion. Nor can it force me to respond. It is neither a wish nor a cause. It is a motive, but a motive given to me by the Other through her weakness. Remember, weakness as weakness is always weak. The weakness of the Other, however, commands me to listen, to answer, and to give goods. Therefore, the weakness of the Other is powerful precisely because it is a gift to my power. It is a gift that arouses my power to be held responsibly. The command to serve is gratuitously given from the weakness of the weak. Her weakness does not lessen my freedom; it consecrates it. It gives my power a power more powerful than the power I use to deceive, the power I use to manipulate, and the power I use to indulge gratification. Her weakness gives my power the occasion for being ethical.

Levinas suggests that perhaps we should not use the word *power* when referring to the weakness of the weak commanding the self to serve. He says that the face of the Other does not have *power* over me, but it has *authority*. However, to emphasize the paradoxical nature of weakness and power, I use the word *power* when I refer to weakness as ethically authoritative, or as commanding power, rather than the demanding power we find in nature or in social oppression. The weakness of the Other as physically and socially (economically, politically, academically, organizationally) weak cannot force me to do anything. But her weakness, always vulnerably exposed to abuse by the advantage of my power, *exposes* me as the advantage-taker, and *appeals* to me with urgency by ethically *commanding* me to *respond responsibly*.

Weakness is powerful for both the weak in her weakness and the powerful inspired by the Other's weakness. It is a gift for both. It is a gift to both from each that binds them not into a totality but in acts of responsibility. The weakness of the weak calls out and consecrates the responsibility of the powerful, and it is the response of the powerful that honors the weakness of the weak, and lends power to fulfill the needs of the weak. The hunger of the man I gave money to yesterday was partially served, and made me more human.

Yet, precisely because these acts of filling needs are responses of ethical responsibility, rather than events of natural or social forces, the partners remain independent. The powerful and the weak retain their separation. Because they are separated, they are able to have an authentic relationship, not a determining causal structure that reduces each to a role, or a mechanistic part of an oppressive unity. The weakness of the weak is authentically powerful because it appeals to the freedom of the powerful to respond. The responsible power of the powerful is authentically powerful because it respects the freedom and dignity of the weak. It gives its power as a gift. It does not reduce the weak by forcing its power on the weak. The man's hunger did not overtake me, nor did my generosity reduce him to a mere object of my generosity. His hunger was the free appeal of a dignified human. My money was a gift of my freedom. We were independent before our encounter; we were independent after we parted. We both kept our dignity as we both contributed to the dignity of the other.

How is the weakness of the weak powerful for both the weak and the powerful?

1. For the Other as *weak*: it is both the source of her ethical command, and also the source of the benefit to her needs.

   (a) The vulnerability of the weak, precisely because it is vulnerable to my violation, is powerful in its command, "Do not do violence to me."

   (b) The need of the weak, precisely because it is not able to force me to respond, is powerful by its ethical call to me, "Serve my need."

The beggar is successful when his vulnerability does his begging. He will likely be rejected when he harasses a would-be giver. The beggar may often be successful by his manipulation, but the responsible giver may still be responding to the destitution of the harasser, in spite of his manipulative harassment. Or, if the giver gives only because of the harassment, we might infer that it is *power forcing weakness*, not *weakness calling forth power*. Ordinances against panhandling may protect against violent harassment, but, when misinterpreted, they can violate "the secret that the strong need the weak," as Vanier tells us, no less than the weak need the strong.

2. For me as *powerful*: being called to serve the weakness of the Other is both the source of my being unburdened of my selfishness and also the source of my powers of authentic understanding, effort, and enjoyment.

   (a) The weakness of the weak Other has the power to weaken my capricious violence as powerful, and calls me to respond, "I will not do violence to you."

   (b) The weakness of the weak Other energizes my abilities, motivating my response to her call, "I will serve your needs."

The weakness of others can break through my tough skin and touch that nerve of responsibility to shock me from my egocentric complacency, which we have described as violent to others and self-sabotaging. The weakness of the weak makes my power *vulner-able* (*vulnus* "wound" + *able* "able," able to be wounded, cut away), able to have my tendency toward violence *cut away*. The weakness of the weak awakens *simplicity* in me. The weakness of the weak commands of me *humble labor*. The weakness of the weak arouses my *patience*. I am moved by *compassion* and *generosity* with gifts. These abilities lie dormant, or misused by me as powerful, until called out. The weakness of the weak is the source of my redemption. The word *redeem* comes from the Latin *redimere* (*re-* "back" + *emere* "to buy"). It is originally the goodness and vulnerability of the Other that saves me, and only secondarily does my good response redeem me. Without these gifts from the weak Other, I remain trapped in my own self-righteousness. My skills are useless when selfishly working for only my benefit. I am repulsive to others as I wallow in my self-indulgence.

THE POWER OF WEAKNESS

Simplicity: The Gift of Self-Skepticism for Attentive Understanding

At the cognitive level of knowing, the weakness of the other inspires my *simplicity*. Simplicity is an *attentive understanding* of the Other so that she can teach me about herself. Her needs awaken me and draw me out of myself. My attention is opened from the outside by the Other. This attention offers me the gift of self-skepticism. Attending to her needs makes me question my self-originating understanding of her. Simplicity is a radical openness to the known unknown. Simplicity is not stupidity. Simplicity is *disinterested commitment to the truth* revealed by the needs of the Other. The simplicity inspired by the need of the Other is a gratuitous gift. It is not an act of an egocentric will. It is nothing I could achieve on my own. I am attentive because the Other's needs and dignity command me to question my own self-interested understanding of not only her, but also of myself, and of other Others. Her weakness offers me the simplicity to place in doubt my own limited perspective and to be taught: to listen, see, be touched by her needs, to search for the conditions that have made her weak, and for the behavior that might help.

Her weakness inspires me finally to become *intelligent: observant* and *rationally thoughtful*. My attention is a focused, but receptive unknowing. The naiveté of my simplicity is not an ignoring, but a desire to know. It is sensitivity, exposure to what it does not anticipate, an openness that suffers the approach of the Other's otherness. It is not blind, deaf, and fearful of the truth. Simplicity is vulnerability to the truth. The wound suffered is the mark of the excising of my self-deception, and, in its place, the truth of the Other can be held.

Simplicity is unburdened of secret schemes and manipulative strategies, ideologies, rationalizations, and techniques that protect my vested interest. These hardened and heavy defenses are designed to protect me from others. But their hardness and heaviness are the burdens of distortion and isolation from reality. These burdens close me off from the truth. The simplicity inspired by the Other's weakness is free of my vested interest that sabotages me.

Humility: The Gift of Self-Substitution for Obedient Service

The word *obedient* does not mean subservient, compliant to another's wishes against both my own and her best interest. Obedience is from the Latin *obedire*, to listen to (*ob* "to or toward" + *audire* "to hear"). Obedience is to authentically listen to and be touched by the needs of the Other and to freely choose to serve her. Obedience offers me the gift of self-substitution. Her command is a gift appealing to me to put my energies at the service of the Other. The humility of obedient labor is not the cowardice of subservience. Humility does not de-energize and render my abilities impotent. The Other's weakness finally commands me to exert effort to accomplish the needed tasks and develop the skills for more work. I am obedient because her needs and worthiness commands me to direct my abilities and energies away from my selfish projects and to work instead to give her the condition to live in dignity. Humility is disinterested commitment to work for others, stripped of capricious self-interest. The humility offered by the weakness of others is a gratuitous gift. It is not an act of an egocentric will. It is nothing I could achieve on my own.

Patience: The Gift of Self-Sacrifice for Compassion

At the affective level of feeling, the weakness of the Other arouses in me *patience*. Patience is expressed in compassion and generosity. The word *patience* is from the Latin *patiens*, from the present participle of *pati*, "to suffer." But patience does not mean "suffering for the sake of suffering." Suffering in itself is useless. Only suffering for others redeems suffering (Levinas, "Useless Suffering," 1988). To be patient is to suffer the worthiness and neediness of the Other calling me to not be violent and to be responsible. The word *compassion* does not mean "to feel pity for," where pity is to have sorrow mixed with disgust for the weakness the weak have brought on themselves. Compassion is from the Latin *com-* ("with") + *pati* ("to suffer"). To be compassionate is to suffer with the Other in order to fulfill the needs of the Other. *Patience* offers the gift of *self-sacrifice*. The Other's needs command me to restrain my tendency for selfish satisfaction, especially my haughty disgust, to put myself in the place of the Other in order to help her enjoy the satisfaction of her needs.

The patience offered in compassion is also not self-denial fueled by self-hatred. If I have self-hatred and am severe with myself with punishment, it is not the patience offered to me by the weakness of the Other. Authentic patience does not make me perversely focus on myself like some innocent lamb sacrificing itself. The temperance of authentic patience is more like a self-forgetfulness, an inattentiveness to my needs because my attention is pulled out toward the needs of others. Authentic patience receives, and it gives. It often errs by exhausting its supply for its own use. But my authentic patience tries to take care to provide for myself in order to reserve strength for attention to others.

Furthermore, authentic patience enjoys good things in the shared celebrations with others, those great and small rituals of honoring the fundamental dignity of each individual human and our connection to each other. The patience offered to me by the weakness of the Other is a gratuitous gift. It is not an act of an egocentric will. It is nothing I could achieve on my own. I receive power in these conditions of weakness, these gifts of *simplicity, humility,* and *patience.* Out of the weakness of the Other, I am unburdened of my complicating and narrowing *obsessions,* exhaustively driving *compulsions,* and destructively decaying *addictions.* I receive the power of relationship by opening myself to the Other. And I receive freedom, power to respond, because that freedom is invested in me by and for the needs of others. To be *attentive* is to receive the power of knowing by understanding the needs of the weak. To be *obedient* is to receive the power of acting by exerting effort for the needs I have heard in the Other's appeal. To be *patient* is to receive the power of feeling by suffering with the Other in trying to satisfy her needs.

So the weak one receives power for her needs by drawing forth my *attentive simplicity,* my *obedient humility,* and my *patient compassion.* My ego-centered self, when weakened by the command of the Other, receives this other-centered power to be responsible. The needs of the weak command me, "Do not disregard me. Do not turn away. Attend to my needs. Especially, do not do violence to me." And I respond, "Here I am, the one guilty of the tendency to selfishness; and, here I am, the one ready to be responsible."

This is how I find myself and my identity, by responding, "Here I am." I understand, at the most fundamental level, *spatiality* by finding my lived spatial location: "Here I am, in this place, facing this needy Other." I can't get out of this space without being irresponsible. If I turn away, I leave the place assigned to me by the call of the Other, the place facing the one who from need faces me.

I understand at the most fundamental level *temporality* by finding my lived temporal location: "Here I am, at this moment of time, being touched by her command." If I delay, if I beg off because of my busy schedule, if I judge that her immediate need at this moment does not have any rights over my present interests, then I have reduced her call to an event in a moment of time easily exchangeable for any other moment of time. Reducing these moments of time to interchangeable events is essentially to *totalize* time, to *annihilate* time. Nihilism is the destruction of distinctions. Destroying the distinction of these moments of the needs of the

Other and my chance to be responsible makes history the inevitable ticking toward meaninglessness, toward nothingness. I can neither turn away nor delay without being irresponsible.

The weakness of the weak evokes in me *self-skepticism, self-substitution*, and *self-sacrifice*. Self-skepticism describes the experience of having my egocentrism questioned by the Other's needs revealed. Self-substitution describes my service put in the place of the Other without displacing her from her spatial and temporal identity. Self-substitution is not pushing her aside; it is putting myself at her disposal. Self-sacrifice describes when my selfish needs, exposed as selfish by the priority of the Other's needs, offers my goods and comfort for her needs. Her command for my self-skepticism, self-substitution, and self-sacrifice invites me to receive the investment of responsible freedom by the needy Other to give her goods in return. The weakness of the Other is the occasion for me to become free from my seductive obsessions, from compulsive habits, and from addictive consumption. Power (freedom) invested in me by others is powerful because it is received from others (its only real source) and used for others (its only real use). Real freedom is received from others. It is not self-made. The self's identity is not self-made. It is found in the response to the needy Other, "Here I am."

The *origin* of the power of the self is not in the self, but in the Other. The *place toward* which this power is to be directed is not in the self, but in the Other. This is the insight of the paradox of the *power of weakness*, that insight inspired into me by the Other. The weakness of the infinitely worthy Other is the *origin* and *intentional direction* of the self.

Seen from this paradox of the *power of weakness*, how, more specifically, do I find the *origin* and *direction* of my *understanding*, that understanding upon which all my other understanding is derived and used? How do I find the origin and direction of my *effort*, that effort upon which all my other effort is derived and used? How do I find the origin and direction of my *satisfaction*, that satisfaction upon which all my other satisfaction is derived and enjoyed? How are choices, success, and happiness experienced from this *original and directed responsibility*? How do I find my identity within this radical awakening to the paradox of the self: that the center of the self is not in the self, but in the responsibility to the Other?

THE ORIGIN AND DIRECTION OF THE SELF

The origin and direction of my *understanding* comes from the Other's revealing the conditions of her needs: the nature of her needs, how to fulfill them, and the abilities to serve, all inspired by her neediness. All other understanding makes proper judgments and appropriate choices for the task of responsibly attending to the Other.

This original and directed understanding can only come as a gift from the needy Other, not from self-reflection, especially from the reflection of a self-righteous intelligence that blinds and deceives itself. Original and directed understanding is only gained by *attentive listening* to the Other: *simplicity.*

Attentive listening is the psukhological condition of Other-centered understanding. The weakness of the Other teaches me about the Other's needs. When I find the Other ignorant about her needs, incompetent to fill those needs, and unable to satisfy those needs, I am pulled out of myself to search for that understanding in order to teach her.

While the call to teach initially exposes me as ignorant of the Other's needs, it opens me to see through the needy eyes of the Other. Confronted by the needs of the Other, I am shaken by a *radical self-skepticism*: the Other is *always-more-than* my understanding of her. She always slips from my intellectual grasp. Her otherness is beyond me. Her infinite otherness is the origin of my simplicity. The horizons of my self-originated and directed consciousness of her is very limited. What a gift is this simplicity!

The Gyges complex (self-centered understanding) is the self-deception that I can hide myself from others and also know them by the power of my own intelligence. Being attentive for Other-centered understanding finds that being *known* by her is the very origin and gift of my self-understanding. When she looks at me, I have the direct experience of being known. This throws me back on myself. The experience of being known makes me become reflective. The content of my reflection is that I am the one who is faced by another who is always-more-than I can know. Therefore, my self-understanding is of the one who originates from the inspiration of the Other. I am not the source of my own self-understanding; the Other is. The claim of independent self-discovery, of being self-made, of being responsible only to and for myself is a cultural and egological myth. It is the product of Western individualism and my own selfishness to want to believe that myth.

The origin and direction of my *effort* is acting with energy invested in me by the needs of the Other. Energy breathed into me, inspires and animates the receptors and sinews of my body to search and provide for the good of the Other. All other effort is to develop personal skills to achieve success in the tasks of serving the needs of the Other.

This original and directed effort can only come as a gift from the needy Other, not as a self-generated and self-directed scheme for my success. Self-generated and self-directed effort becomes manipulative, abusive and alienating to others, and ultimately self-defeating. Original and directed effort can only be gained by being animated, by being *obedient*, by doing *humble* labor.

Being *obedient* is the psukhological condition of Other-centered effort. The weakness of the actions of another (her failures) commands my help for her success. When I find her failing in her efforts, I am called to exert effort to repair her failures and guard against further loss.

This call to serve another exposes me as ultimately helpless in absolutely ridding her of failure and suffering, but commands me to do what I can. "I am not called to be successful, only to be faithful." Mother Theresa has given us this powerful mantra. The failure of the Other commands me to search for ways to help and to exert effort to do what I can, despite the possibility of failing to relieve her suffering failure. Confronted by the neediness of the Other, I am struck by a *radical self-substitution*: the needs of the Other command me to set aside my own interests and to put my labor in the place of the Other. This self-substitution is a task I cannot accomplish in the sense of replacing her, because she is *always-more-than* the place she takes up and the effort she gives. The substitution to which I am called is to be of service to her in her dignified identity. She holds her own space and time. I do not push her out of the way. I am committed to her retaining her place and time by substituting my service where she needs help.

She calls me to serve beyond my ability, yet I cannot shirk my responsibility. This *humble labor*, this simultaneous shock of both inadequacy and irreplaceability inspires the gift of *self-substitution*. Her command to me to serve commands me to deny myself and exert effort despite my deficiencies. In this way, I find my true self to be the one called by another, with inadequacies exposed, to effort exerted, hopefully for her needs to be satisfied. What a gift to me is the opportunity for *humble labor*!

The Zeus complex (ego-centered effort) is the self-deception that the origin of my possibilities and restrictions lies in myself and not in others. This self-deception tries to convince me that no command from outside can move me. It tries to convince me that I am not accountable for the negative consequences of the exercise of my abilities, because those consequences are the justifiable cost for my culturally guaranteed individual freedom.

The origin and direction of my *enjoyment* comes from my desire for this Other's goodness, not for my satisfaction but for hers, always respecting the otherness of the Other. All other enjoyment is the satisfaction of my needs in order to love the love of life so that I might offer it to the Other.

This original and directed enjoyment can only come as a gift from the needy Other, not from my acquisitive and envious interest in her. Original and directed enjoyment is only gained by disinterested desire for the good of the Other, by being *patient* with the Other, by being *compassionate* and *generous*.

Being patient grows out of the psukhological condition of Other-centered satisfaction (her satisfaction). Her weakness, her suffering, evokes from me feeling for her, compassion and generous giving of whatever of myself I can to help release her from suffering. The alleviation of her suffering is the only usefulness of my suffering. Levinas makes it clear that suffering in itself is useless.

This call to provide for the Other by giving up my own comfort is a command that cannot be totally filled. I sacrifice to give, but my sacrifice is never enough to alleviate all her suffering. She is *always-more-than* the conditions I am able to manipulate in order to reduce her suffering. Confronted by the neediness of the Other, I am struck by a *radical self-sacrifice*: I must give up not only my things and comfort, but also my self-definition as a successful caregiver. Her suffering is always beyond my reach. I can offer her human company, place her in safety, and give her health care, bread, and money; but I cannot guarantee her satisfaction and happiness. I cannot reduce her satisfaction to the result of my actions. She is infinitely beyond my grasp.

This radical sacrifice, this simultaneous shock that I am powerless to totally rid her of suffering, yet inescapably challenged in the call to work to rid her of suffering can be the gift of compassion. The Other's command to me to give to her calls me to sacrifice even to the extent of abandoning my bloated notion of altruistic concern. This "poverty of spirit," as Johannes Metz calls it (1968), offers me my true self: exposed as a self-indulging ego by the suffering of the Other, yet commanded to provide comfort for her, though ultimately unable to relieve her suffering, and, with this poverty, sharing with her and enjoying what we have together, this is the *I*. What a gift is this *patience*!

While, on the one hand, my Narcissus complex (self-centered satisfaction) is the self-deception that I am the origin of my own satisfaction, and therefore have exclusive claim to it; on the other hand, patience, compassion, and generosity recognize that my purest enjoyment comes from the needs of the Other being satisfied, the deepening of my desire. My deepest enjoyment is paradoxically the expression of gratitude for the needs of the Other being filled and for my finding myself able to respond, honestly facing my poverty and yet offering it to the Other.

Levinas calls my inescapability from the call of the Other *proximity*. Ordinarily, we use this term *proximity* to indicate the spatial location and distance between things. Levinas uses it to indicate the *always there* of the Other, which is the ground zero of space. He calls the radical otherness, the incessant escape of the Other from my grasp, *transcendence*. Ordinarily, we use this term to indicate how I can rise above my baser self to a higher self. Levinas uses it to indicate the *always beyond* of the Other, which is the ground motive for my rising above my baser self.

The psukhological experience of the Other as simultaneously *always present* and *always absent* is the basis for our existential anxiety. Since Kierkegaard and Heidegger have defined the notion of *anxiety* as the experience of the uncertainty of the self about itself and its inevitable, yet unknown, time of death, I will use Levinas's terms *insomnia* (no rest, no escape from responsibility), and *honor* (celebrating the rights of the Other over my own). But it is precisely this *insomnia* and this *honor* of the Other that save me from egological death in life.

HOW THE WEAKNESS OF THE OTHER EMPOWERS THE SELF AND EMPOWERS THE OTHER

The neediness of the Other is always there calling me and is always beyond my understanding, effort, and satisfaction. This *proximity* and *transcendence* of the Other holds power over me. On the one hand, the Other's *proximity* is the never-ending presence in both time and place of the Other. Of course, there are times when I have no other person spatially near me. But the Other is present even in her absence: I am *obsessed* with the Other (Levinas, 1974/1981, p. 86). Levinas does not mean a neurotic obsession, but an ethical obsession. I can never conclude that I have done enough, that I can turn away from her, that I can forget about her. I may have done all I can, but I cannot judge that my efforts have done enough. *Proximity* commands *insomnia*, figuratively, or rather ethically, if not literally. I cannot rest, take a vacation, or release myself from the responsibility to be ethical. Of course, I rest, vacation, and relax to keep myself able. But I can never rest from being ethical. Being ethical is not a psychological or spiritual state in my soul. It is a relationship to concrete others.

On the other hand, the Other's *transcendence* is the never bridgeable otherness of the Other. Of course there are times when I have *intercourse* with the Other, in the many ways that word is used: talk to, share with, compete against, organize with in a system incorporating both of us, as well as "make love to." But the Other is always absent in her presence: she is separated from me by her freedom; I am separated from her by my freedom. I cannot comprehend, control, and consume her. She is always *other*, always worthy by her own independent existence, always requiring my service. Levinas does not mean her oppressive mastery taking advantage of my neurotic servility. To honor is to ethically respect the Other's independent dignity, her rights over me. Her dignity as a person remains, even when she exercises vicious cruelty against me or others. Of course, her behavior is not dignified, not to be honored. But she still has needs to which I am called to attend. I can never conclude that her selfishness cancels her dignity, which is based on her human existence. I can never conclude that her needs are within my power to fulfill. I may have done all I can, but I cannot reduce her and her needs to my understanding, labor, and enjoyment.

Transcendence inspires *honor*. I cannot dismiss the Other from my responsibility to be responsible to and for her. I can and must judge her behavior, stay clear of her abusiveness, and develop my own skills and enjoy my life; but I can not unethically judge her, defend myself against her, individually develop myself, and enjoy my greedy indulgence.

The unresolvable ambiguities of her *proximity* and *transcendence*, and my *insomnia* and *honor* of the Other is a power that exposes my egocentrism to myself, and gives me attentive self-understanding and an understanding of her that is simple. It releases me from my self-sabotage, and gives me obedient labor that is humble. And it breaks my addictive indulgence, and gives me patient enjoyment with the other. Authenticity is found in acknowledging and committing to the paradoxical combination of the *proximity* and *transcendence* of the Other.

Hearing the Call to Responsibility, I Am Identified as the One Assigned, and I Respond

The weakness of another exposes me and questions my own power not only over her, but also over myself. My centering, my self-reflecting, my self-directing, my self-nourishing cannot authentically come from my self-initiated understanding, effort, and enjoyment.

The recognition of the narrowness of the horizons of my understanding cannot come from my own willful constituting consciousness. If I am at all simple, open to the reality beyond my narrow understanding, it is because I am given simplicity by the Other. The recognition that I am using my skills only for my success cannot come from my own willful behavior. If I am at all humble, laboring for the good of others, it is because I am given humility by the Other. Placing limits on my satisfying my own needs at the expense of others cannot come authentically from my own willful providing needs. If I am at all patient and compassionate, sacrificing my pleasure for others, I am given compassion by the Other.

When she says, "You do not understand," and I interpret her *exposure* of my narrowness as an attack, "You are stupid," and respond with defensiveness and critical judgments, I will have lost the opportunity for self-reflection. When she says, "That is not helpful," and I interpret her *exposure* of the limits of my skills as a criticism of me, "You are useless," and detach myself from any effort to act responsibly, I will have lost an opportunity for self-directing to improve my abilities for helpful work. When she says, "Don't selfishly take it all," and I interpret her *exposure* of my not sharing as calling me greedy, "You are a repulsive pig," and further selfishly indulge myself to regain my feel-good self-image, I will have lost the opportunity for self-nourishing to love life.

Although the origin of my *simplicity, humility*, and *patient compassion* is from the worthiness and needs of the Other, and although I often tend to misinterpret her questioning my understanding, skills, and satisfaction, still, discovering my limitations requires my own self-denial. It seems such a foolish paradox this universal religious saying, "I center myself by denying myself." But it is not foolish. It is wise. I am decentered when, thrown back upon my conscience, I deny my selfish claim to the arbitrary use of power, and truly centered when I find my real power in the obligation to use the abilities invested in me by the weakness of the Other to give power to her weakness. Her *proximity* and *transcendence* revealed by her facing me has power over me, but it is a blessed power. Her face, revealing her weakness, awakens me to my true self. I am a self when denying myself in order to be other-centered. My self-denial is a gift from the Other. It is not the product of my intelligence, my exertion of effort, and my generosity to satisfy with my magnanimous self.

I find myself when I respond, "Here I am. I have misunderstood, misused you, and taken pleasurable advantage of you. Now I am here to understand and teach, to discipline myself and serve, and to give and celebrate with you." This is the self-skeptical, substitutional, and sacrificial responsibility that defines the very I-ness of the I: the one who cannot rest and is called to honor others.

SELF-REFLECTION: ATTENTIVE UNDERSTANDING BY BEING QUESTIONED

At the level of knowing, my self-reflection originates in the face of the other questioning me. My independent self-questioning is susceptible to an obsession with myself. In authentic self-questioning, I do not so much question myself as I am questioned by the neediness of the other. My self-reflection comes from listening to her questioning. She opens up horizons unknown to me. When my knowing is emptied of self-righteousness and intellectual arrogance, I am opened for self-understanding. I am attentive. Listening to her questioning gives me the gift of simplicity.

SELF-DIRECTION: OBEDIENT SERVICE BY BEING COMMANDED

At the level of acting, my self-directing originates from the ethical command of the weakness of the Other. To be commanded is to have the

Other breathe into me the meaningful motivation to labor for her good, to be obedient. The self commanding itself is susceptible to a compulsivity that is motivated by ego-centered success. I do not so much command myself as I am commanded by the neediness of the Other. My direction is being obedient to humbly refine my skills, and labor for the success in service of others.

SELF-NOURISHMENT: GRATEFUL GENEROSITY BY BEING IMPOVERISHED

At the level of feeling, my self-nourishing originates from being impoverished by sacrificing for the needs of the Other. To be impoverished is to give up my possessions and consuming, in order to give to the Other. On the one hand, when I impoverish myself by willfully imposing temperance and austerity on myself, I am likely to indulge myself with self-righteous self-sacrifice. Self-sacrificial asceticism denies the inherent goodness of the enjoyment of things. This can lead to denying goods for the neediness of the Other based on some self-generated conclusion that the good is not good for the Other. On the other hand, when I nourish myself by being impoverished for the sake of the Other, I do not so much nourish myself, as I am nourished by the sacrifice for the neediness of the Other. My self-nourishing is being compassionate to the Other.

Listening to the Command to Be Responsible,
I Give Self-Disinterested Service

For absolute authentic service, my interest must be disinterested. The dignity of the Other must be recognized as absolute (*ab-solvare*: washed of), cleansed of any vested interest by me. My service is for the sake of the Other. Service to others is susceptible to being motivated for some secret benefit to the server. Attending to the Other's absolute dignity is recognizing her value to be independent of any value to me, and evaluation by me. The Other's absolute dignity is infinite dignity freed from any judgment by another.

The Other remains infinite, always more than . . . that which is within the grasp of my serving. In a way, as a server, I always fail. I can never fulfill the Other's needs. The successful outcome of my service can never totalize her dignity. Furthermore, as a server, I can never completely absolve, wash away my own self-interest. My inherent egoism keeps me from this ideal. Recognizing that I am not called to be a *successful* servant, only to be *faithful* to the Other, demands the sacrifice of myself as the one with inherent tendencies to be obsessed with knowledge, success, and enjoyment, and therefore to be a meddling intruder. I am called to respect and guard the Other's place. My response is "Here I am! Use me!" This retreat from imposing self-claimed power over the Other invests power in the Other. When the self gives freedom to the Other, the Other is truly served.

Listening to the Other offers her the chance to discover on her own an understanding of her needs. Before I can teach her about the conditions and skills to achieve the satisfaction of those needs, I must listen to her expressions of need. Self-disinterested listening is authentic service because it is founded on the weakness of the Other who calls me in the first place to question my irrelevant instruction, and, in the second place, to listen attentively to the expression of her needs, to remain awake and to honor her words.

Self-willed listening to others can become a condescending insensitivity, patronizing with an air of superiority. Authentic listening is being open to the Other's expressions, an openness founded on my admission of ignorance. This unknowing of her, this simplicity I have received from her can invest in the Other, now liberated from my self-righteous judgments of her, the power to understand herself and her world because she can safely reveal herself. Her self-understanding, inspired by my acceptance of her, opens her to seek information from me that might help her. This is genuine teaching!

Obedience, as self-disinterested serving, offers the Other the chance to safely exert her own effort to help herself, and helps me to exert my own effort to serve her self-help efforts. To admit my failures in helping, with improper skills, is humbling for me. My labor is humble when I provide assistance without quitting the effort to honor and support the Other's plans and work.

Self-willed obeying is susceptible to ego-centered manipulation, claimed to be for the good of the Other. Or my obeying may be a subservience, motivated by my laziness, or my cowardice to risk failure, or my inordinate need to be needed by the Other. Authentic obeying consists in having my freedom invested in the humble labor to fill the Other's needs for her sake. My humility, now liberated from my arrogant manipulation of her, invests in the Other the power to act on her own and become successful. Her self-help, inspired by my willingness to help her rather than to use my skills on her for my good, can seek my help. This is genuine helping!

At the level of feeling, to serve, I must not give only out of my abundance, that which I do not need. I must give more than what I do not need. I must feel the loss to my body, sacrifice my satisfaction. I must offer my body to be appropriated as a means to satisfy her needs. The only means to satisfy a need is the sacrifice to another's body. This is my only authentic gift. Levinas uses the image of the parent who takes the bread from her mouth and the milk from her body to give to the child. The story of a woman and child in Turkey trapped for days under the rubble from an earthquake is seared in my memory. When her child became weak from loss of nourishing fluids, the woman cut the end of her finger with broken glass for the child to suck her blood. Both survived! This is a model for all service. Helping hurts.

If I hurt myself for the sake of hurting when I help, I have missed the point of helping. I must help not just until it hurts, but until I have done whatever I can for the good of the Other, which may or may not be beyond the point when it hurts. When I give my body I become susceptible to a perverted enjoyment in the pain of sacrifice, especially in the glory I expect for being a sacrificing helper. This is inappropriate because my ego, distracted by my self-image as a sufferer, does not attend to the Other's needs. Her needs are unfulfilled, because I did not give of myself for her sake.

Her continuing needs face me and expose me. When my inappropriate gift is exposed to me, I can authentically nourish real compassion, and real generosity. My compassion, now liberated from the decadent seductions of my inattentive and inappropriate gifts, invests in the Other the power to nourish herself by the enjoyment of real goods. This is genuine providing!

Cooperating by Vulnerably Trusting the Other

Trust means more than hoping to receive a reciprocal support from the partner. Trust means I am open to receiving no return benefit. Cooperative trusting acknowledges, (a) that I am elected to be responsible for the Other before understanding her needs, before I choose to be responsible, and before I am certain that I will receive a benefit, (b) that I am even responsible for her responsibility, and, (c) that, in filling her physical needs, I find my spiritual needs.

In cooperation, I and the Other cannot succeed alone, yet I cannot demand reciprocity. Trust, not demand, is absolutely essential for successful cooperation. Trust provides the Other the freedom to be responsible, and of course the freedom to be irresponsible. It is fundamentally a risk for me, founded on her weakness calling me, in the first place, to question my need to demand equal reciprocity, and, in the second place, to join up with her in a common effort to help each other. My service must be absolved (washed clean) of the demand to receive return contribution. Without my demand, the Other is absolutely free to cooperate and serve me in return. Her weakness questions my arbitrary and calculating power to demand equality. Her questioning weakens my ego-centered demanding, allowing her to freely serve me in return. This is the beginning of cooperation in relationships. If cooperation dissolves into scheming for equality and reciprocity, it has lost its foundation of trust, and its power to gain shared success. Trust includes the *hope* that the partner will reciprocate, but does not demand and undermine the trust.

When the Other is given the gift of my vulnerability by trusting rather than demanding, she, in return, can invest in me the freedom to further trust her. My role in being vulnerable when I invite her to trust me to use my freedom to trust her does not take away her role of responsibility. Without my taking my role in being responsible even for her responsibility, she cannot take her role in being responsible. Self-responsibility can only be inspired in an atmosphere of trust. The authentic power of cooperation comes from the mutual trust of each other. Suspiciousness and demanding sabotages cooperation. When I respond to the call of another, I am responsible to and for her. I am called to join her and to be invested with a freedom by her to be exercised for the common good. My response is: "Here I am; I am ready to give in cooperation even at the risk of not receiving an equal share, in order for you to trust me and fulfill your responsibility. My trust of you is how I am responsible for your responsibility."

DIALOGUE: ACKNOWLEDGING THAT I AM CHOSEN

The dialogue in cooperative knowing is conversation. In conversation, the speakers *converse* (*con-* "with or together" + *-verse* "turn"). We *turn over together* the topic of our dialogue in our talk by a mutual self-skepticism, self-substitution, and self-sacrifice by looking at the topic from each other's perspective as well as our own. We each really listen. We step out of our own perspective in order to enter the experience of the Other. We really speak *to* the Other, not just *about* the topic from our biased position.

Speaking begins by being spoken to. Even if the Other does not open her mouth, her face speaks to me prior to my understanding of the topic to be discussed. The origin of conversation is in the appeal expressed in her face as it faces me. Her independent worthiness and neediness questions my tendency to prejudge her. This is the first signification (meaning), the first *saying* between us, her invitation to me to speak and to speak truthfully. She calls me to be self-skeptical, to set aside my own interests, to be genuinely interested in her and the topic of our conversation. My expression of disinterested interest acknowledges my ignorance about what she is about to say and is my openness to her. Before any words are spoken, before I know what is to be spoken about, I am chosen to responsibly listen. I must express my responsible trust of her prior to the Other's explicit request.

As the Other sees and listens to me trusting her as she calls me forth into conversation, she can trust my appeal to her to enter into a real dialogue. We can lose ourselves in a real dialogue. The mutual bond appeals to my self-substitution. On the basis of this mutual trust, the back-and-forth questioning and answering probes and discloses the world. Levinas makes it clear that speaking in dialogue is primarily a speaking *to* the Other, and secondarily a speaking *about* the topic. Even less is it a speaking *from* my narrow preknowledge. This speaking *to* is one way I am responsible for the Other's responsibility. I am responsible for inviting her to responsibility. My expression of trust invites her to trust. I speak *to* her. Then we can speak *about* the topic.

Conversation as learning together is powerful because the weakness of the Other calls me to question, on the one hand, my initial understanding of her needs, and therefore genuinely ask about them, and, on the other hand, to listen in trust to her speak of real concerns. In speaking to me of her concerns, she deepens her understanding of her own needs. When she calls me out of myself and appeals to me to understand her, then she invests freedom in me to be a genuine listener about her world. She listens to me appeal for understanding of her needs, and she is then freed to disclose her needs for my understanding.

Her weakness through her lack of understanding disarms me and calls me to respond to her ignorance as simplicity rather than stupidity. Her simplicity calls my self-righteous judgment about her ignorance into question. My acknowledgment that her ignorance is a simple unknowing allows her to trust me and therefore teach me about her real self. The origin of understanding is not in my powerful knowledge, but from her in her simplicity calling me to understand. I know myself and my world when I respond, "Here I am. I am here addressed, called to understand, and to respond."

COLLABORATING: RESPONSIBILITY FOR THE OTHER'S RESPONSIBILITY

As I have stated above, trust is being responsible for the Other's responsibility. This claim can be misunderstood. It appears to be the condition for codependency. But, being responsible for the Other's responsibility is not to take over the Other's responsibility from her by demanding and *manipulating* the Other, and thus making her dependent. When I demand, I do not allow her to be responsible for herself. My responsibility is to appeal to her to be responsible, not to take from her her responsibility. There are several situations in which we can find the truth of Levinas's bold statement that I am responsible not only for the Other, but also for the Other's responsibility.

When I act collaboratively with another for our common good, I depend on her, but trust her. I recognize my need to contribute my part, and trust the partner to contribute hers. I must not pull back my trust and begin calculating the amount of her contribution in order to be assured that I am getting my share and not getting cheated by her. I guard against her mistrust of me, not by a mistrusting guard, but by trusting her, by recognizing that I am responsible not only for my responsibility, but also for the Other's responsibility.

In some collaborative efforts the tasks assigned to each partner overlap. Either could do any part of the task. In this situation I continue to work on any part because it attends to the task and its completion. I am responsible for all the parts, trusting the Other to work on some, but recognizing my responsibility for even the Other's responsibility, the Other's assumed part.

When my partner must be responsible for some part of the task, because I cannot do it, I am further responsible to urge and trust the partner to responsibly do my part as well as hers. If this collaboration is a genuine cooperation, I cannot demand, but only appeal to the partner to contribute. I am responsible for the Other's responsibility.

Certainly, at times, cooperation breaks down. Partners renege on agreements, or adopt a style of competing to assure at least equal reciprocity in costs and benefits. When the partner fails to uphold her part, it is her inherent dignity, despite her cheating me, that calls me to question my own arrogance in judging her by suspiciously placing limits on my trust. I must forgive and trust. She can only cooperatively contribute in an arena of trust, rather than suspicion. Therefore I am responsible for her responsibility.

I recently spoke to a group of contract managers of a large manufacturing corporation that held many subcontracts. They described the *legal* need to write contracts that cover any possible loopholes the other's corporations may find. But they further described the *psychological* need to develop the conditions of trust between themselves and the contract managers of the subcontractors. In face-to-face meetings, each legally represents their companies. But it is the face-to-face trust, the vulnerability, the appeal to the trust and vulnerability of the other that make a contract work.

We receive power for cooperation when we respond, "Here I am. I am here to help and to be helped. My absolute trust is essential to our collaboration. This is how I fulfill my responsibility even for your responsibility."

Sharing involves the Other-centered division of goods when I allow the loss of my share of the limited goods to the Other for her enjoyment, trusting, but not demanding, that she will share with me in return. The Other may or may not give enjoyment back to me. When I trust the Other to share, I am giving her the freedom to share the goods in return, or not to share them. Sharing is powerful because the Other's need calls me to question my need for my due share, to give her freedom to enjoy the goods, and to open the possibility to receive or not receive the Other's gift in return. If I demand the equal division of goods, I suspiciously accuse her of not intending to share and withdraw the freedom I am obliged to give her in my trust.

When others call me out of myself and appeal to me to trust them in return, then they invest freedom in me, and I can freely trust them. When, rather than remaining in my selfishness, I respond to their call to be trusted, their call questions my tendency toward selfish decadence. They call me to consent to, be grateful for, and even enjoy the suffering I sacrifice as the price of trust when it is suffered for their good. I do not masochistically enjoy suffering for the sake of suffering. I enjoy the enjoyment of the Other provided by my suffering. Suffering in itself is useless. Only suffering for the needs of the Other is redeemable. It provides my spiritual need. I have one spiritual need upon which all my other spiritual needs depend. That spiritual need is to get out of my self-deceiving, self-defeating, and self-destructive selfishness by responding to the needs of others. Only their needs can call me out of my selfishness. Striving, out of my own self-serving need, to get out of my selfishness is self-righteousness. I depend on others, not only for my own physical needs, but especially for my spiritual needs.

I enjoy life, and I live in happiness with others when I respond, "Here I am. I am here to share and celebrate together." My desire for the goodness of the Other, sacrificing my enjoyment, absolved and cleansed of my egoistic interest, can only be filled with absolute trust.

Competition by Challenging for the Good of the Other

As *mutual trust* is the essential ingredient of cooperation, so *mutual challenge* is essential to competition. To challenge is to test the abilities and effort of the Other for the sake of the Other. The power of competition lies in helping the Other improve by urging her to test her skills and effort against my skills and effort. This Other-centered challenging is delicate. On the one hand, I must seek out the Other's weak skill in order to challenge her to strengthen this skill. On the other hand, if I take advantage for myself of her weak skill, I may not be helping her strengthen her skill.

Her vulnerability calls me to question my compulsive tendency to win, to gain power over her for the sake of power rather than for the sake of challenging her to strengthen her skill. To genuinely test her, I must offer a genuine challenge, no half-hearted reluctance out of a false sense of kindness. Her request for my challenge calls me to try to out maneuver and resist her skills and effort. Only by meeting a real challenge can she test her skills. I must really try to win.

If motivated by my ego-centered drive to win, my challenge would be an effort to escape my responsibility to serve the Other by challenging her skill. To compete, I must cooperate with the Other, trust the Other to use my challenge to improve her skills, but not try to beat me so that I am no longer a challenge. To trust the Other, I must make myself vulnerable to being out maneuvered by the Other. This is her gift back to me: a challenge for me to improve.

Authentic competition is a delicate and generous gift given to each other. Its delicacy is so frequently broken. The lure of the prize and of a magnified self-image too frequently replaces the generosity available in competition. As we saw in chapter 5, bickering, cheating, beating, grasping the prize destroys competition.

DEBATING: TESTING THE OTHER'S KNOWLEDGE AND COMMITMENT TO TRUTH

Debating is serving the Other by challenging her misunderstanding. To test another's understanding is to hold it up to the light of evidence from the reality of the world. It is not to compare it with my understanding. The task is to seek truth, not to seek a superior position. While self-centered debating tries to convince the Other of my position for my advantage, Other-centered debating helps the Other understand reality as the world presents itself. Challenging for truth is paradoxically weak because it does not use personal or rhetorical arguments to convince; it does not use power. When I debate, I risk the possibility that I might be proven wrong by evidence. Challenging for truth is, however, paradoxically powerful because the weakness of the Other calls me, on the one hand, to question my need to outsmart competitors, and, on the other hand, to search for the truth with her in order to bear witness to reality as it shows itself. Achieving this goal, understanding the world as it is rather than holding an error is powerful in judging and deciding.

CONTESTING: TESTING THE OTHER'S SKILLS AND EFFORT

We can certainly recognize the power of challenging the skills and effort of others. Without being put to the test, skills never develop and deteriorate. If the test is experienced by the Other as my effort to reduce her skills only for the sake of my individual advantage and her suffering, then the primary good of the contest, which is interpersonal respect, is lost. The word competition (*com-* "together" + *-petere* "to seek") means "to strive together." Sports provide classic examples. When the compulsion to win is greater than the respect for the Other, then the value of the game is lost. Other-centered contests are powerful because the Other's weakness calls me to question my need to win by whatever means, and simultaneously to fully challenge each other to exert effort together to improve skills and effort.

Genuine competition contributes to the growth of the community. With improved skills, members of the community can better serve. Competition is naturally entertaining to observers. Watching skillful competitors striving together by seeking out each others' weaknesses and guarding their own draws the admiration of onlookers for the courageous risk-taking of the participants, and the sheer beauty of human behavior. Nearly everyone enjoys sports. But when the mutual challenge for mutual service is replaced by egoistic motives to win at all costs, nearly everyone gets disgusted.

MARKETING AND SHOPPING: TESTING THE OTHER'S TASTE AND GENEROSITY

Since consuming is not simply fueling a physical system, but is even more the enjoyment of filling our needs, we can compete by testing each other's taste for enjoying. By challenging the Other's taste, urging her to rise above mere fulfillment to enjoyable satisfaction, I improve my taste in the challenge, and ultimately we give each more enjoyment. The end of mutual challenge to enjoyment is to celebrate together our gratitude for the goodness received. If my challenge to the Other's taste is motivated by an ego-centered effort to enjoy the goods alone and to flaunt my affluence in a showy display of expensive taste, then I do not serve the Other, nor myself.

Improving each others' habits of consuming provides the basis for us to share with other Others. We have a deep human desire to enjoy together, expressing shared gratitude. Enjoyment is the embodied experience of gratitude. Enjoyment is the experience that the good enjoyed came not from me, but from elsewhere. Enjoyment is both my individual experience of the goodness of the good, and the recognition of dependence upon the good and others who provided this good. Enjoyment is gratitude. We can enjoy together the good we have given by investing in each other the power of good taste. This is celebration. Celebration is the expression of mutual gratitude. Giving to another is the natural expression of celebration, the expression of the gratitude of having received what I do not deserve. Celebration is honoring again and again the surprise, the awe in receiving the goodness of the good. Celebration is proclaiming to another the goodness of the gifts, and the desire to share this goodness with the Other. A celebration is Other-centered, not self-centered, not conspicuous consumption. It is honoring goodness by sharing goodness. Goodness is so good, it must be given away.

Leadership by Honoring and Serving Others

When others have invested power in me to use to decide and direct the organization, then my ego-centered power is weakened and my Other-centered power is strengthened. They have placed their trust in me. They have made themselves vulnerable to my misuse of that power. Their chosen weakness, however, calls my individual power into question and assigns me as the one who must use my invested power for their good. This assignment is to protect them from abuse by others, to provide them the knowledge they need, to assign behavior to fit with other contributing members, and to justly distribute benefits. My *authority* has the invested right and power to *author* the events and activity of the organization. This power has been divested by the individual members of the organization to consolidate it for its efficient service. When leadership power is used for that purpose, then it is powerful.

The power of my leadership is powerful precisely because it is received from others to be used for others. As an authority, I have taken upon myself the burden of responsibility for all those under me. I must be sensitive to the needs of those others. This sensitivity requires a passivity that radically open me to the expression of needs. I must listen. As authority I must make decisions concerning the good of the whole that may not be the best for specific individuals. Likewise authority must make decisions that benefit the needs of individuals so that of their neediness does not cost the group. To the call of my subordinates, I respond, "Here I am, the one invested by you with corporate power to bear witness to your work, to invest you with power to do your work, and to celebrate our shared success."

EVALUATING AND PLANNING: BEARING WITNESS TO THE DIGNITY OF OTHERS

The face of the Other proclaiming her fundamental dignity speaks the first truth. As a leader, I must bear witness to that truth. The dignity of the individual Other has been made vulnerable under the power of authority she and others have invested in me. Her vulnerability calls me to question my tendency to abuse this vulnerability, to plan and decide for my ego-centered advantage. Her investing power in me has called me to be individually weak, not to use my skills for my gain, but to use them for the good of the organization and each member. I must use my power to protect all who have invested their power in me.

MANAGING: INVESTING POWER BACK INTO OTHERS

Setting up an authority, rather than each member's retaining their individual power, avoids the likelihood of chaos in the event of a threat from outside the group or from internal strife. Authority provides efficiency. Authority guards against abuse. Authority exerts effort to stop the misuse of members by either fellow members or by members from competing organizations. The power received from subordinates, making them vulnerable, must be used to honor them by protecting them. Their weakness calls me to question my cowardice against abusers.

Authority directs the behavior of the individual members according to the evaluation and planning available to that authority. There are multiple systems of organizing corporate structures to balance efficiency and morale, the enjoyment of honor by the authority. I cannot describe the many new forms of power-sharing in management being developed in society. My simple understanding is that there are often imbalances between efficiency and morale. The compulsive drive for raising productivity and profit has sacrificed the honor due to both workers and consumers. My interest in the study of authority in organizations is only to emphasize the role of continual service and honor of the members by those in authority.

DISTRIBUTING BENEFITS: GIVING AND CELEBRATING

The authority must justly distribute the goods of the common effort. There is great power in the distribution of benefits. Goods are good because they fill needs and are enjoyed. Since goods are essentially common property to be used to fill needs and to enjoy satisfaction, the authority must distribute them justly, giving a preference to suffering of the weak. Their weakness reveals that their investment of power into the authority has been a greater sacrifice to them than those who gave less because they had more.

The weakness of the Other calls me to question my tendency to be apathetic in the face of the suffering of others and, on the other hand, to give needed goods to those suffering and celebrating with them.

CONCLUSION

This is the power of weakness. This description reveals the psukhological experience of facing others. Although infinitely distant from me (transcendent) and infinitely close to me (proximate), they do not restrain my freedom, but invest freedom in me. Their weakness limits my capricious and self-directed freedom. Others inspire me to a more authentic freedom in the service of others. While the others' weakness remains weak, this weakness is the source of their power. While I retain power, their weakness invests this power into knowledge, action, and satisfaction for their good.

The method used in this chapter was a *phenomenology of responsibility*. Responsibility backs me into insomnia by never letting me rest from that responsibility to honor the dignity of the Other, to attend to her needs, to labor for their satisfaction, and to celebrate our enjoyment of the goodness of the world. Humbled by the neediness of the Other, I *listen to* her expressions of need, especially because of my tendency to abuse, and I *respond* to her "Here I am. I am the one who has heard your call. My power is from you to be used for your good. I cannot shirk my responsibility."

PART IV

The Paradox of Community

Interlude

Social Justice Based on Radical Altruism

Peter raised his hand from the back row.

This philosophy of Levinas and your Other-centered psukhology are too idealistic. This is not the way people behave. It would, of course, be a wonderful place to live if everybody respected the rights of others above their own. But unfortunately the world is populated with egocentric people, and therefore everyone else must pull back and adopt a cautious attitude, a self-protective set of habits to keep from being taken advantage of. We can trust an inner circle of friends and family, but, if I read Levinas right, these close acquaintances and relatives are not radically *others*. They are more like the *same*. I can respect the rights of my neighbors over mine because I'm sure they won't use their rights to abuse me. Levinas is great for describing people in pockets of the trusted few. He is not helpful for the larger issues of social justice.

There are three ways with which I respond to this objection. First, Levinas, having lived through the Holocaust, knows well the evil people do to each other. His awareness of the tendency toward violence is always present in his descriptions of the utopian situation where saintly people act responsibly toward each other. His is a meta-ethical philosophy that tells us outright that holiness is better than viciousness. Al Capp, in his marvelous comic strip of the mid-century, portrayed Mammy Yokum giving Lil Abner the straightforward advice that "good is better than bad." Levinas offers us a hagiology (the study of saintly behavior). His is a description that assumes that kind and generous consciousness, behavior, and affect is better than selfishness that hurts others. Psychology also should be able to describe the ways people act when they respond to the goodness of others with regret for their own selfishness and with kindness toward others. Mainstream psychology, as an *egology*, seems to describe people as if their motives were only self-interested.

161

My second response to objections to *radical altruism* is that our progressively cynical culture urges us to be suspicious of descriptions of Other-centered responsibility. We have developed personal and institutional habits of being critical of others, of claiming to be victims of others and suing them, of competitively taking advantage of others, and of grabbing and hoarding consumer products for our enjoyment at the expense of others.

My third response is that Levinas's Other-centered philosophy does not urge the self to become a victim of others and stoically accept their dominance. It is his radical altruism centering the self in the Other that places limits on the self's skepticism of itself and deferring to the Other. His radical altruism places limits on the self's substituting itself for the Other in ways that would make the self a victim. His radical altruism places limits on sacrificing enjoyment for the Other out of some self-centered ascetic motive.

I will take these three responses in order, first using Wyschogrod (*Saints and Postmodernism*, 1990) to help with the importance of the postmodern study of saintly lives, then using Sloterdijk (*Critique of Cynical Reason*, 1987) to help describe our modern cynical mindscape, and finally using Burggraeve (*From Self-Development to Solidarity*, 1985) to describe the limits to self-sacrifice.

THE APPEAL TO HAGIOLOGY: EDITH WYSCHOGROD

Nobody disputes that there is a real distinction between ethical belief and ethical action. Nor does anyone dispute that ethical behavior is learned mostly by observing and imitating other good people. We admire people who give of themselves for others and we often try to copy their actions. The selfish behavior of others attracts our attention in the opposite direction as what is to be avoided. We teach our children to look up to generous models and to associate with kind friends and peers. We tell them about examples of good lives that even seem to be beyond imitation. Hagiology, the study of saintly behavior, is learned mostly by observing what we call special models and reading about or watching on video the lives of ethically heroic people. Thankfully, our good models are still most often parents, grandparents, siblings, neighbors, other teachers, coaches, counselors, pastors, and others. We learn in church and school about models like Abraham, Buddha, Confucius, Mohammed, Jesus, St. Francis, Lincoln, Mahatma Ghandi, Dorothy Day, Martin Luther King Jr., Archbishop Romero, Mother Teresa, Eli Weisel, and Jean Vanier. We are taught admirable behavior in the stories from history, biographies, and fiction. Whether all the models held out to us were never egocentric, always altruistic, is not the point. There is in society a concerted effort on the part of teachers to teach ethical behavior by holding up idealized examples of Other-centered people.

Edith Wyschogrod, in her book, *Saints and Postmodernism: Revisioning Moral Philosophy*, recommends that we return ethical studies to reading the narratives of saintly lives. The study of ethical theories, she says, does not often change behavior for the better. Wyschogrod claims there are two problems with the traditional study of ethics.

> One difficulty connected with moral theory is the gap between the theory (even when it is a theory about practice) and life. The aporia between theory and practice is particularly apparent in modern theories from Hume to the present. (1990, pp. 3–4)

> A second problem is the failure of recent moral theories not only to settle moral questions but, more significantly, even to agree upon terms of moral disputes. This is not a lexical failure but the result of the heterogeneous philosophical background claims that govern attempts to resolve disputed questions. (1990, p. 4)

While little overall practical result can be reached by reviewing, comparing, or contrasting the abstract theories of moral philosophy, the lives of good people have always inspired other people. Wyschogrod suggests, for learning about ethics, employing narratology (the study of narrated lives both real and fictional) especially hagiography, the lives of the saints. She cautions, however, that hagiography has been problematic. The typical "lives of the saints" have been too often sentimental distortions attempting to inspire readers to piety but not necessarily to authentically holy behavior. The narrated stories of saints often try to convert readers to a denomination or to a theology. Sometimes biographical accounts of special people are used to rhetorically argue church politics. Conservative factions try to describe their past leaders as saintly while their holiness seems derived from their social philosophies rather than from personal humility, service to others, and self-sacrifice.

Although we must be cautious of the motives of the authors, the lives of models, those stories, whether put in the language of mythical figures of primitive tribes or in the language of modern heroes, still move us toward ethical behavior more than do theories.

Fictional accounts frequently get to the essential characteristic of what Wyschogrod calls the saintly style. She says that what is central to the lives of saints is their "recognition of the primacy of the other person and the dissolution of self-interest" (1990, p. xiv). She defines the saint more explicitly as one whose adult life in its entirety is devoted to the alleviation of sorrow (the psychological suffering) and pain (the physical suffering) that afflicts other persons without distinction of rank or group or, alternatively, that afflicts sentient beings, whatever the cost to the saint in pain or sorrow. (1990, p. 34)

In her text, Wyschogrod adds to her formal definition the claim that "[o]n this view theistic belief may but need not be a component of the saint's belief system" (1990, p. 34). We can easily find examples of these extraordinarily inspirational fictional characters. For example, Graham Greene gave us an ethical model in *The Burned Out Case* in the character of a formerly renowned architect he named Querry. Despite others calling him a saint, he claims to have no God, denying any of his behavior to be admirable, denigrating his accomplishments, living in despair of his own life, escaping to the heart of Africa from an explicit ego-centered life, spending his days bandaging lepers, caring for the most powerless, and designing and building a simple but functional hospital. In the end, he is accused falsely and assassinated by a self-righteous religious fanatic. Greene did not have Querry, this "saint," convert to any religious belief, despite the efforts of the priests, nor did he have him find value in any of his own actions or virtues. He was simply a good man who devoted himself to the alleviation of sorrow and pain of others without distinction of rank or group, whatever the cost to himself in pain and sorrow. His was disinterested interest.

Tarrou in *The Plague* (1948) is an equally admirable character. Albert Camus, himself as atheist, created this fictional atheist who had no ulterior motives beyond helping others. Tarrou's interest was truly altruistic, caring only for the well-being of others.

Most saints, although they may be grounded by some religious faith, describe how they were moved to action by the needs of others rather than for fulfilling some dogmatic conviction. It is this quality of disinterested holiness that leads readers who do not belong to the denomination or theology to be inspired by the lives of saints. Christian saints such as St. Francis of Assisi, St. Ignatius Loyola, and St. Martin de Porres have become models for people who may know little of their religious beliefs, but who admire their sacrifice for others. The lives of saints are consistently read not because of their beliefs, but because they were radical altruists.

Levinas's philosophy is not a hagio*graphy*. Although he comments on characters from the Bible and on Talmudic readings in his religious works, he does not narrate stories of saints in his philosophical works. Yet it is a hagio*logy*. He tells us the essential characteristics of holiness: a desire on behalf of the Other that seeks the alleviation of the Other's suffering and the fulfillment of the Other's needs for enjoyment. He does not ask us to turn our attention to his abstract statements to find the motives to act ethically. He asks us to turn to the face of the Other, to respond to the call of the needs of others in their powerlessness, to recognize *the primacy of the Other person and the dissolution of self-interest.* Our individual lives are moved to ethical behavior by being face-to-face with the individual lives of others in need. For Levinas, holiness, not self-interested moralistic behavior, not a theory about moral behavior, is authentic ethical behavior.

The argument that the idealism of Levinas's philosophy is an unreachable utopia is an empty criticism. Of course, in its purest form, a society populated by citizens inspired to perfectly self-disinterested interest in the exclusive good of others is unreachable. But it is a vision of what a completely humane society should constantly be trying to be. It is, according to Burggraeve (1985), "an *effective* utopia, since, as an ethical demand, it continually stimulates man to surpass his egocentric society and not to halt before the already realized heteronomous social structures" (p. 126).

Levinas's philosophy as an ethical ideal is itself fragile, vulnerable to the attack of other ethicists. His meta-ethics does not rest on muscular rational ideas. It does not convince by logic. It is not based on primordial principles independent of any human persons. Its first *idea* is not a principle; it is the nonintentional, passively received idea of *the infinite dignity of the Other revealed to us by the face of the Other.* Levinas's work does not exhort us to do good. It tells us to open the eyes of our eyes, to listen to and be touched by the face of others who will tell us to do good. It is fragile because our response rests on opening ourselves to the needs of others and choosing to respond. The call to be responsible comes from the Other not as a causal demand but as an ethical command. A command can so easily be interpreted cynically to justify our irresponsible response.

THE CYNICISM OF IDEOLOGY: PETER SLOTERDIJK

As a hagiology, the description by Levinas of what inspires ethical behavior is fragile because postmoderns have become suspicious of any moral philosophy. We think we have had too much moralism. The modern moral crusaders, with their religious, political, economic, educational ideologies, have for so many modern observers paradoxically inspired distrust rather than acceptance. Moral ideologies frequently attack competing moral ideologies. The self-righteousness of many ideologies inspires distrust in their own righteousness because of their arrogance. We moderns are too smart to be taken advantage of by the hypocrisy of moralists. We are too skilled in achieving success to be held back by the dictates of those who set up ethical principles and ethics review boards. We are too rewarded with the good things of life to be distracted by the claims of those who appeal for a more just distribution of these good things.

The second response to student objections to the *too much*-ness of Levinas's philosophy is that, because of too much moralism from ideologies, too much skill in getting around rules and regulations, too much comfort in our personal situations, we moderns are prone to cynically place Levinas's philosophy into the ranks of just another moralistic theory. We are well practiced in criticizing moral systems.

Peter Sloterdijk, in *Critique of Cynical Reason*, describes how modernity is characterized by a diffuse but pervasive cynicism that has invaded all levels of our society. I will follow his suggestion (1987, pp. 101–103) to distinguish two opposing kinds of cynicism. We can begin one with the letter *k*, as in *kynicism*, connecting it to the original Greek, which had a *kappa* in its alphabet but no letter *c*. Given its historical roots in ancient Greek philosophy, we can call the necessary habit of suspicion and criticism *kynical*. We can spell the second kind with the letter *c*, as in *cynicism*, connecting it to the modern tendency to be arrogantly critical, manipulative, and self-indulgent. *Cynicism* is the corrosive effort of modern self-righteousness that has contaminated much of our academic, political, economic institutions. A cynical general public is abused by and criticizes these institutions.

Clearly we need to be *kynically* observant and critical of the corruption and hypocrisy of others, especially those who hold some official or charismatic power. The nihilistic abuse of public trust demands constant watchfulness and systems to remove abusive leaders from their positions of power. While philosophical nihilism is the denial of any basis for truth, the garden variety of nihilism can be found in the coffee houses of the sixties and seventies, and now around the water-coolers on the eighty-seventh floor. Modern public nihilists deny the legitimacy of all principles, values, and institutions they have not benefited from. The practical nihilism of corrupt and hypocritical public figures is the leveling of all values except their self-interest. In an open and democratic environment where power depends on the trust invested in leaders by subordinates, those with that power must give the appearance of interest in the public good. Yet appearances of morality and nihilistic hypocrisy need to be exposed. Cynicism needs to be challenged by kynicism.

Let me continue this discussion of the distinction between *kynicism* and *cynicism* with the story of the original kynic, Diogenes of Sinope, who lived around 350 BC. Legend has it that Diogenes went about Athens during daylight with a lantern. When asked why, he said, "I am looking for an honest man." He was a critic of the intellectual snobs, the politically powerful, and the self-indulgent of decadent Athens. He ridiculed other philosophers and announced his own ethical beliefs, not by writing tomes, speaking in the forum, and seeking student followers, but by living simply and acting on his beliefs. Diogenes taught by refraining from pontificating, refusing to collaborate with the politically powerful, and living in poverty. Alexander the Great, hearing of Diogenes' fame, sought him out to learn from his wisdom. This great Greek general promised to grant Diogenes any wish. Sunbathing at the time, Diogenes asked, "Stop blocking the sun."

He was called the "dog" of Athens. The word *kynic* comes from the Greek word *kuon*, meaning "dog," or from *kunikos*, meaning "doglike" or "currish." He lived, out in the open, the simple animal life and in a sense barked at and verbally bit those who showed hypocrisy. His lived philosophy joined the happiness of the satisfaction of his simple needs together with penetrating observation and uncomplicated but profound thought.

Although we need modern *kynics*, we do not need isolated hermetic characters contributing only negative criticism. Like the old Greek who, with cheeky but dogged pursuit of truth, used sarcasm to criticize the hypocrisy of the arrogant, the manipulators, and the greedy, we need to expose the insolent self-righteousness of modern cynicism and to bear witness to those who generously devote their lives to the good of others.

The modern cynical style we see taking advantage of our supposed contemporary enlightenment, our refined efficiency, and our affluent enjoyment is burdened with suspicion. As things get better, they seem to get worse. There is widespread discontent in modern society. Sloterdijk's point in *Critique of Cynical Reason* is that while many moderns living in this Age of Enlightenment consider themselves to be "with it," they have only been seduced by the notion that "knowledge is power," and have thus lost what it means to be enlightened, to have knowledge for the sake of knowledge, not for the sake of power. Their *enlightenment* justifies their cynical criticism of the fools who have brought on the problems about which they are discontent. They have been seduced by available beliefs and theories that conveniently serve the vested interest of their positions of power. But their sophistication has not brought them happiness.

Sloterdijk claims that they are not really enlightened: "we come to our first definition: cynicism is *enlightened false consciousness*" (1987, p. 5). Enlightened false consciousness seems to be an oxymoron. Generally, we define false consciousness as claiming what are known to be errors to be true. But besides simple errors that are based on logical or perceptual delusion and can be corrected relatively easily, there are also ideologies.

According to Sloterdijk, an ideology is a "persistent, systematic error which clings to its own conditions of existence" (1987, p. 15). Sloterdijk, the historian, tells us that in the modern age ideology is power. While many moderns living in this age of efficiency claim to be "highly effective people" through the use of sophisticated technology, particularly the technology of personal and social organizational behavior, they have too frequently only been seduced by technologies that promise efficiency, but do not save either time or energy. Individuals look around and find their organization is better off, but that they are not better off. They are working longer hours and enjoying it less. Heather Menzies make this very clear in her recent book, *Whose Brave New World?* (1996). At the level of behavior, people find the system of the organization taking advantage of their work, rather than their being able to take advantage of the system. The competition between the individual and the larger organization (business, government, school, church, even family) cynically justifies the individual in efforts to *use the system* for his or her own advantage.

Moderns, in this age of enjoyment, also try to convince themselves that they are, or soon will be enjoying life. If we really believe that we could attain the images offered by advertising, which is precisely what the advertisers hope to convince us, we could hope for a paradisiacal existence. The cars in the television advertisement sweeping around the beautiful country road look as if they are about to take off into heaven. But moderns have too frequently been seduced by the enticements of sophisticated marketers to consume junk. Sloterdijk says that their cynicism "is that modernized, unhappy consciousness. . . . They are well-off and miserable at the same time" (1987, p. 15).

With these insights from Sloterdijk, and using the three levels of the psyche (cognitive, behavioral, affective), let me define modern *cynicism*. At the cognitive level, *cynicism* is the ideological justification for being certain about social realities and being contemptuous of the ideas and behavior of others. At the level of behavior, cynicism is taking advantage of others by "using the system" all within the rules of the game of individual competition. At the affective level, *cynicism* is the greedy gratification of our wants because the ego justifies its just deserts for being good. Of course, the cynic believes, those who suffer want didn't earn rewards and do not deserve them.

At the cognitive level, cynics claim to be penetrating observers of hypocrisy and to be astute critical thinkers, and they are bound by a duty to correctness. They consider themselves to be especially perceptive of the psychological characteristics of others. They have read or watched a lot of pop psychology, which fills the bookstore shelves, pervades talk-show discussions, and enlightens the insights of some fundamentalist preachers of politics and economics as well as religion. Enlightened cynics know how women feel and men feel, how older people think and youth don't think, what motivates buying behavior, leisure activity, and sexual encounters, how to raise children, how to get along with co-workers, how to make lots of money, and on and on. The air waves are filled with ideological justifications of the vested interests of these self-appointed pedagogues, demagogues, and psychogogues. The preachers of modernity have sophisticated rhetorical skills to seduce followers into their own cynical mindscape.

At the behavioral level, while criticizing others, especially those who run *the system*, cynics find ways to use *the system* for their own benefit at the expense of others. They manipulate rules and regulations by finding loopholes and exceptions while expecting others to be held to the letter of the law. When society depends more on regulations than on ethical relationships, it invites cynical opportunism.

At the affective level, while criticizing others and using the system, cynics justify their own indulgence of pleasure as a reward for their self-initiated productivity. Modern advertising has convinced masses of people to reward themselves, while it has simultaneously convinced them that they must be discontent with what they have.

Let me back up a bit and briefly outline the history of modernity and the crashing down on us of a postmodern world. Mary Jo Leddy, in "Formation in the Post-modern Context," describes this world:

> [T]he modern world . . . was a world shaped by the Enlightenment, by a confidence in the human capacity to know the world through science and to shape it through technology. It was a powerful secular vision which exalted know-how and can-do and which promised liberation from the determinism of nature and the strictures of tradition. It celebrated spirit—the spirit of human inquiry and inventiveness. It promised progress. (1991, pp. 7–8)

She goes on to say, however . . .

> My own view is that the vision of modernity was definitively shattered not by thinkers but by the events of twentieth-century history. Auschwitz, Hiroshima. These two events have become challenges we are still grappling with. If this is what technology can do, can we believe in it? Can we still believe in progress in the face of such barbarism? . . . Environmentalists have signalled the destruction to the biosphere which has resulted from the unfettered use of technology. Feminists are questioning the mode of domination which has developed along with the mod-

ern vision. . . . A younger generation no longer believes that it
will have a better life than that of its parents. The twin mythologies of mastery and progress, integral to the modern vision, are
in doubt. (1991, pp. 8–9)

Now the outline. If we ask, using the three levels of the psyche, what
we think we gain and from what do we think we are liberated through the
advancements of the modern age, we can state, what modernism has
achieved, what power has gained and what weakness has avoided:

Psychological levels	What modernism has achieved	What power has gained	What weakness avoided
Cognitive:	Scientific knowledge	Enlightenment, understanding	Ignorance, misunderstanding
Behavioral:	Technological development	Efficiency, success	Inefficiency, failure
Affective:	Production and distribution of consumer goods	Enjoyment, comfort	Suffering, discomfort

I do not claim that science, technology, and goods are inherently bad
for us. It is the illusion of their promises and our resulting cynicism that
shatters us.

If we have gained so much good and done away with what we found
so bad from earlier dark and primitive ages, then why have we become so
cynical? Without an accompanying self-skepticism, self-substitution, and
self-sacrifice, the triple powers of enlightenment, efficiency, and enjoyment can undermine their own value. We are shocked by the unanticipated consequences of becoming obsessed in the ideologies of the day in
place of simple understanding. We are horrified by the development of
tools of mass destruction of peoples and the earth and of compulsive techniques of institutional manipulation in place of the smoothing out of the
rough edges of life. We are distressed by our addictions to junk food, junk
television, and junk gadgets in place of the celebration with others of our
shared happiness and genuine prosperity. We have found that obsessive
certainty is paradoxically ignorant. Compulsive control is paradoxically
failed behavior. Addictive consumption paradoxically brings suffering to
ourselves and to our neighbors in need.

On the one hand, there are more and more ethical regulations being
adopted and enforced in government, business, education, church, family, and entertainment. There are also more voluntary efforts to follow
moral requirements. There are the new "virtuecrats," "socially responsible investing," demands for a return to moral education in our schools. I

recently read that the Marine Corps is adding another week to boot camp to instruct the recruits in ethical behavior.

On the other hand, there is a constantly growing disrespect and distrust of government, business, schools, churches, families, entertainment, and the military. As the call for morality rises, so suspicion of hypocrisy deepens, and cynicism widens. There is a dialectic between *cynicism* and *hypocrisy*. They seem to be codependent. The cynic obviously needs the hypocrite, without whom the cynic would have no one to criticize. It is obvious to the cynic that hypocrisy should be obvious to everyone if they opened their eyes.

Just as much, the hypocrite needs the cynic. The hypocrite must believe that all others are hypocritical as well as himself; this is his cynicism. He justifies his hypocrisy based on his suspicion of others. If the hypocrite thought there were only kynics, critics who themselves lived exemplary lives, then the hypocrite could not so openly practice his hypocrisy. The nihilism of both hypocrites and cynics amounts to the same in both. The cynic's self-righteousness convinces him that he comprehends the hypocrisy of others by finding they fit the categories of his ideology. His certainty is based on his belief in his ideology. His comprehension and certainty justify his reducing others and manipulating them to serve his righteous ends. His self-indulgence is justified as reward for his righteousness.

Sloterdijke is a very astute reader of modern cynicism. But he offers us no hope because he offers no serious description of a *radical altruism*. His *kynic* is as trapped in his ego as is his *cynic*.

THE LIMITS TO ALTRUISM: ROGER BURGGRAEVE

Only a radical altruism can place limits on that kind of self-skepticism, self-substitution, and self-sacrifice that is ego-centered and therefore destructive of authentic community.

The philosophy of radical altruism seems counterintuitive to students when it is first introduced to them. It seems to demand *too much* of the self in submission to the Other: *(a)* Too much skepticism of the self's own knowledge would seem to abandon any hope to understand truth. Truth would be relativistic, relative to the need to serve the Other. *(b)* Too much substitution of the self into the service of the Other would seem slavish. *(c)* Too much sacrifice of the self's own needs would seem masochistic.

So a third response to student objections to Levinas's astonishing philosophy of responsibility to and for the Other, to his radical heteronomy, and to a psukhology that describes cognitive, behavioral, and affective events motivated by the altruistic desire for the good of others, is to find within this philosophy reasons to limit forms of altruism. I have depended on Roger Burggraeve's book, *From Self-Development to Solidarity: An Ethical Reading of Human Desire in its Socio-Political Relevance according to Emmanuel Levinas* (1985) for articulating Levinas's limits to altruism. His references to many of Levinas's untranslated works has given me access to these notions of limits on altruism. He quotes Levinas from *Du sacre au saint* (p. 21):

> "While in principle the Other is infinite for me, one can to a certain extent—but only to a certain extent—limit the scope of my obligations." The interjection "to a certain extent" means that the responsibility itself can never be rescinded, but only limited: we are not concerned here with the defense of my rights, but with the limitation of my duties. (1985, p. 107)

So, on the one hand, a philosophy of radical *egology* (the center of the self is in the ego) begins with the first principle that the ego has rights over others. It must use this principle of self-interest to justify any limitation to its own egoism in order to explain responsible behavior. For *egology*, responsibility to others must follow responsibility to the self. Since acts of responsibility begin in the ego (as all acts in an egology begin in the ego), the ego must be the source even of any limitations placed on the ego.

On the other hand, contrary to an egology, a philosophy of radical *heteronomy* (the center of the self is in the Other) begins with the first principle that Others have rights over the self. This first principle is actually not a principle but an experienced fact of the radical otherness of the Other revealed in the face of the Other. Levinas customarily simply referred to the fact of the Face when pointing to the revelation of the otherness of the Other. From this fundamental fact of the Other's rights having a priority, the self must use reason to find justifications for exceptions to altruism. Since, in a radical altruism, the origin of responsibility is from the Other, not from the self, any limits placed on service to others must be derived from this primary ethical responsibility to others.

Authentic altruism cannot be explained by a radical egology. Egology can only describe egocentrism. While egology in principle reduces all human events to self-interest, radical altruism does not claim any behavior is inevitably caused by other-interest, but that the Face of the Other calls us out of our tendency to egoism to act responsibly toward others. Authentic altruism that places limits on its own altruism can only be explained by a radical heteronomy that includes all others. Burggraeve explains Levinas's point:

The third party introduces a tension, or even a contradiction in the responsibility presented above (in the text) as so pure and elevated. The third party sets limits on my infinite responsibility for the one Other: the hunger of the proximate Other is an absolute demand which tolerates no delay, hemming-and-hawing or "measured" answers, but rather conscripts all my possibilities and sources of help—"only the third party's hunger can limit its rights." (1985, p. 107, quoting Levinas, *Difficile Liberté*, 1964, p. 10)

The following are justifications for placing limits on altruism based on the primacy of the call to responsibility by and for all others.

1. First I would like to stress Levinas's pre-ethical concern for the self. He beautifully describes how the self and its happiness are good. A person with an identity with self-understanding, self-developed skills, and healthy habits of self-nourishing is a good in itself and sought for its own sake. Burggraeve points out how Levinas recognizes there is legitimate concern.

for my own self-development situated on the level of my "natural" dynamism of existence. This . . . clearly is pre-ethical and thus is motivated from within the very self-development: it is self-development from within and *because* of self-development (or one's happiness). (1985, p. 108)

The experience of gaining knowledge, accomplishing personal success, and satisfying its needs establishes the separateness of the "I": the I-ness of the "I", the self-identity as a separate person. The "I" cannot serve the needs of others without experiencing its separate identity. The self identifies itself over time and place,

a. By having a clear understanding of its motives, abilities, memories, and anticipations, both pleasant and painful, and of its relationships to others, and by confidence in its knowledge so that it can alter its self-understanding when proven wrong

b. By developing a structure of habits and dispositions that bring success, and, when it fails, the ability to change to improve its actions;

c. By not only satisfying its needs to nourish itself to carry on, but also by enjoying the satisfaction of its needs and loving its life.

Self-identity does not *have* cognitive, behavioral, and affective habits the way it possesses its owned goods. The I *lives from* its understanding, actions, and enjoyment (Levinas, 1961/69, pp. 110–14).

The "I" is founded on its experience of "Here I am! Confident in knowing what I know, doing what I do, enjoying what I enjoy." Self-identity is not to be negated, cancelled out, found inherently wrong. Certainly self-identity is "called into question," bracketed by the needs of others, set aside for the sake of others. But self-identity can only be called into question for the sake of others if it is experienced as a good. The priority of the Other's needs over those of the self does not render the self's needs unworthy of filling. Radical heteronomy expressed by the face of the Other commands the self to put its cognitive, behavioral, and affective identity in the service of the needs of the Other.

2. The self is limited in its service to others because of the limits to the self's possibilities.

> The fulfillment of my responsibilities in accordance with my powers and possibilities requires a limiting of the Other's unlimited right and of my infinite obligation with regard to him. (Burggraeve, 1985, p. 107)

Others and their needs are *always beyond the comprehension* of the self; their acts are *always beyond the control* of the self; and their satisfaction is *always beyond the provisions* of the self. If the self were able to totally understand, manipulate, and satisfy the Other, the Other would be an object or product of the self. But the Other is always beyond the reach of the self. It is not the limitations of the ego per se that limits the self. The possibilities of the self are limited because of the infinite otherness of the Other.

3. The self can not serve the good of another by letting the Other take advantage of the self and violate the self.

> The original inequality of my infinite responsibility for the Other is corrected by the fact that I too fall under Other's responsibility. (Burggraeve, 1985, p. 110)

While the Other's needs call the self to question its self-priority, if the Other abuses the self, this abusive behavior would not be a good for the Other. The self must not contribute to the harm of the Other by allowing the Other to be violent. Restricting the Other's behavior can be a service to the Other.

4. The self must not serve the Other if that act would violate yet another Other (a third party).

> If I effectively fulfill my responsibility for the third party, perhaps I do my neighbour injustice; and if I direct my attention to my neighbour, I undoubtedly fall short in my duties to many third parties. (Burggraeve, 1985, p. 106)

When acting in a society of others, the self must respond to conflicting needs between two or more others. Although the self cannot compare one Other with another Other, because they are both beyond the comprehension of the self, the self often must compare these incomparables and choose between other Others. Justice begins when the self must weigh the rights of others competing for the services of the self. The results of weighing rights of others will always limit the altruism of the self for others.

5. The self must set aside time, energy, and interest in order to develop itself to have something to offer to others.

> Levinas forcefully states that this limiting of responsibility not only can but *must* be accomplished. . . . [I]f I have nothing which I can offer the Other, I cannot fulfill my responsibility. (Burggraeve, 1985, p. 107)

The self must, *(a)* grow in knowledge, *(b)* refine skills, and *(c)* nourish its strength, by satisfying needs as preparation for responsibility. The self must limit its altruism in the service of others in order to develop its own knowledge, ability, and happiness in order to be a helper.

6. The self must be cautious that its *good works* toward another are not used by that other to abuse other Others.

> [T]he *meaning* of my deeds no longer coincides exactly with what they are intended to be. They reach further: they receive an "objective" meaning, which is not enclosed in the subjective intentional meaning. Thus my deeds can bring about an injustice which I did not intend. Levinas characterizes this as *social fault*. (Burggraeve, 1985, p. 101)

Generous gifts and actions toward another may be turned into a means of violating the rights of other Others, and even abusing the very one to whom the self gave the gift. The "I" must limit its altruistic giving of gifts if those gifts will likely harm others. The difficulty is, as Levinas says, that the results of a person's *good works* are most often beyond the control of the worker once it leaves his/her hands. For example, the money given to someone might be used to spend on substances harmful for themselves or another. The hard work a person gives to a company might empower that company to act unjustly against others. Nevertheless, the self must try to avoid this *social fault* when it can be anticipated.

7. Given that we are always in situations of multiple others with many third parties, the "I" is always an other for the Other and the third party.

> Through the presence of the third party, I and the Other become like the Others, i.e. their "equal." Or rather: we become each oth-

ers' "like-neighbours." We stand on equal footing with one another. . . . The third party introduces symmetry in the nearness without, however, eliminating the difference, i.e. the ethical non-indifference or responsibility. Equality constitutes our "co-existence" ("co-presence"): we are all "together-in-one-place," we are "one-with-another" without differences of level, that which makes "reciprocity" possible. (Burggraeve, 1985, p. 110)

The self must uphold the model of the good citizen for social justice, which is founded on equality and reciprocity. Setting an example of injustice that allows the other to abuse the self would sabotage the call to social justice. This example of injustice could be used by still others to justify their exercise of abuse toward other Others. The I must support the institutional structures established to guard the rights of others, including the self. The self must assign responsibilities to others even when those assignments benefits the self, if those assignments benefit the social justice of the community. The I must limit its sacrifice if that sacrifice would undermine the society and state that are constructed to preserve general justice.

8. There are a few psychological reasons to limit the skepticism, substitution, and sacrifice of the self. The I must not simply try to escape responsibility by claiming itself to be unknowledgable, incompetent, or unmotivated. A claim of modesty in knowledge, skill, and needs is too easy an escape.

9. The I must not seek a kind of perverted passive-aggressive or masochistic enjoyment of self-humiliation by claiming, (a) stupidity in understanding, (b) failure in effort, and (c) a victim suffering from my own foolishness. This kind of perversion may be seeking sympathy from others. It may be a neurotic pleasure-from-pain syndrome.

In summary, radical altruism commands the self not to serve others for the purpose of serving the self. Altruism is the service of the Other and of others.

With these reasons to withhold the total sacrifice of the self for the Other, based upon Levinas's philosophy of radical heteronomy within the community of multiple others, we can now turn to chapter 7, The Power of Community.

CHAPTER SEVEN

The Power of Community

The community's responsibility for the needs of individuals is based on each individual's responsibility for the Other, for other Others, and for the community.

At the 1993 debate held at the New School of Social Research in Manhattan between a representative of the Cato Institute, a conservative think tank committed to libertarian principles, and Amitai Etzioni, a founder of the communitarian movement, I sat in the audience in wonder. I witnessed what seems to be an unbridgeable gap in political philosophy between *individualism* and *communitarianism*. While individualism has shaped most of the history of American culture, communitarianism has a strong history and is presently trying to place some limits on the negative effects of the liberal use of freedom found at the center of individualism.

Markate Daly says that individualism rests on this philosophy:

> [E]ach person has a unique identity defined by a subjective consciousness, forms and carries out projects that unfold in a personal history, holds an inalienable right to pursue this life plan, and follows universal principles of morality in relationships with others. (Daly, 1994, p. xiv)

Individualism places the *individual* at the center of social/political/economic life. In individualism's extreme form, community is only a conglomerate of individuals. The rights of the free individual is the first principle of the philosophy and practice of liberalism. Individual good is the bottom line. Individual autonomy defines the person.

Communitarianism, on the other hand, is a new, postliberal philosophy of political thought. It could only grow out of the liberal tradition of established democratic practices in a liberal culture. Daly tells us the foundation of communitarianism rests on the philosophy that as a member of a community, each person belongs to a network of family and social relationships and is defined by this membership, and each person seeks personal fulfillment through participation in the evolving social structures of this community, finds personal liberty in an expanded self-development cultivated through these activities, and honors a traditional complex of agreed-on commitments. (Daly, 1994, p. xiv)

Communitarianism places the *community* at the center of social/political/economic life. In the extreme, the individual has rights given them only to serve the good of the community. The welfare of the community is the first principle of this philosophy and practice. The common good is the bottom line. Community membership defines the person.

The philosophy of Levinas offers a third alternative. While his is an individualism that stands firmly on individual responsibility, it is also a communitarianism in that the individual's responsibility for the good of all others is the basis for the common good of the community. The "I" cannot shirk its responsibility for others by arguing that those others do not belong to the same family, tribe, community, constituents of authority of the "I." Although the "I" must compare individuals, in order to judge and choose what contributions need to be made first and under what conditions, all others, simply as human, are worthy of service.

Although Levinas's philosophy of radical responsibility can be considered communitarian, the community does not have priority over the individual. The individual is not called to turn her/his freedom over to a state or any other authoritarian body. Rather than being denied, freedom is liberated by being invested in the individual through the call to responsibility by and for others. The individual is freed from his own capriciousness by the call to responsibility. Choice is called to a higher form of freedom than capriciousness. The community is bonded by individuals protecting the rights of others rather than by a supreme leader or by the grip of vicious competition for self-interest. This kind of individualism/communitarianism of Levinas, described in the Interlude, is indeed a utopian vision. However, it is no more idealistic than the alternative utopian vision that claims that the community will naturally thrive if each individual is responsible only for her/himself and that self-interested competition between individuals is a force of nature that raises the quality of life for all.

We need to articulate how each is responsible for all others. If, at the conclusion of part III, we were to end the description of the relationship between the self and the Other, we would have a shallow vision of not only the self's role in the society of multiple others with its organization of institutional structures and practices, but we would also have a thin understanding of the self's role in relation to the individual Other.

So far, in our reflections in the previous chapters, social interaction has been a coupling of two: I and the Other. But defining society as the conglomerate of individuals and couples misses the fundamental character of society. Social institutions and their structures would be only the accumulated habits of behaviors between individuals. If the face of the Other represented only itself, then social living would be but a series of dialogues between the self and individual others.

The face of the Other is indeed the concrete Other confronting me, accusing me of the tendency toward violence against her rights, and calling me to be responsible. Individual responsibility for the proximate individual Other is the central ethical experience. The face of the Other is *proximate* in two ways. The immediate Other is proximate both, (1) as closer to me than any other person right now, always calling me to be responsible, and also, (2) as closer to me than I am even to myself: "the center of the self is in the Other, not in the self." I am more responsible for the Other than for myself. The Other has rights over me.

But the face of the Other expresses more than the presence of a single other person calling for my immediate responsibility. Besides being proximate, the face of the Other is also *distant*. The immediate Other is paradoxically distant in two ways: (1) as always beyond my comprehension, control, and consumption, no matter how much I think I know her, influence her, and enjoy her, and also (2) as always beyond me because she represents all others, in all places, at all times. She is humanity. It is not only her unique characteristics, her personality, or her membership in a particular group that I am facing. I am facing her universal humanity. Her face faces me not only particularly but also universally. Her accusation of my tendency to violence accuses me of being violent toward other Others as well as toward her. Her call to me to be responsible is a call for me to be responsible for everyone, not just her (Levinas, 1981, pp. 157–62).

As a prototype, when we can look at a love relationship with another, I find this Other has relationships to other Others, family, friends, workplace and neighborhood associates. Although the two of us try to achieve an exclusive situation, at least for a while, secreted behind doors and curtains, lowered voices, and privately meant glances and gestures, the others of the beloved can never be completely forgotten, or considered outside my responsibility. The beloved has parents, siblings, neighbors, friends, work partners, many others with whom she is related. She represents them. They are always there through her.

This is especially brought to light when I seek forgiveness and apologize to the immediate Other on those occasions when I have violated her rights. My violation of the Other spreads beyond the realm of this immediate Other. Since the Other represents other Others, my behavior has an effect on others. Since I cannot undo my actions that violated her, I can only ask the Other to forgive my intentions, and try to make restitution to her. Although she may forgive me, she has little control over the influence of my behavior on those other Others who have been affected by my injury to her. I not only cannot exclude myself from responsibility to other Others when I give and serve the loved one, but I certainly cannot exclude myself from responsibility to those I have hurt by hurting her.

Although the model of natural ecology, describing how every event affects every other event, helps us understand society as an infinitely interconnected ecosystem, we must deepen this notion with the notion of infinite responsibility. Our responsibility extends to every other because they are all infinitely worthy. Ethical responsibility goes beyond the notion of ecology, the balance of nature. My responsibility to other Others is founded not only on the possible effects on them when I interact with the immediate other, like a series of chained interactions. My responsibility is founded also on the fundamental dignity of every human person. I do not owe to the Other only because she owes to another, who owes to still another, who owes to yet another, and therefore links me to those distant others. I owe to all others because they are independently worthy of respect. I may only reach them through the immediate Other who mediates between me and the other Others or the social institutional structures and processes mediating between myself and the other Others. However, I am responsible to and for all others.

So the social order not only extends my accountability because it spreads my violations, it also offers me the means to extend my responsible service beyond my immediate, or proximate, reach. The face of the Other represents humanity through the structures of social institutions. Without the social order, with its far-reaching institutional structures and processes, I have only limited means to carry out my responsibility to those beyond my narrow milieu. The personal bank check I just wrote will not reach hungry people in a Third World country, but my contribution will go through a complex system of economic and political structures and provide them help.

Because my generosity eventually reaches Somalia, it will not reach Rwanda, or Bosnia, or the victims of a natural disaster in another state, or the soup kitchen down the street. Yet I trust that my neighbors' checks will reach those I cannot reach. Society reaches, or better, I reach through society.

PHENOMENOLOGICAL METHOD: COMMUNITY
COMMUNICATES AND ASSIGNS RESPONSIBILITIES

Let me quickly review methods. In chapter 3, assuming an egological perspective, I described the power that we individuals identify as our own power. The phenomenological method for reflecting and describing was to *disclose* and *declare* the phenomenon as it presented itself to us: power is powerful, and power empowers itself. Power is disclosed when I, the ego, declare, "Here I am. I am the center of myself. Take notice of me, because I empower myself." I assume all others are like me.

In chapter 4, still from an egological perspective, I described weakness as the ignorance, laziness or cowardice, and discontent of an individual. Because weakness, by its nature, is experienced negatively and attributed to the fault of the individual, the phenomenological method for reflecting and describing was to openly *expose* this weakness and *accuse* the other individual of her weakness.

In chapter 5, adopting a psukhological perspective, I began to attend to the paradoxical, to that which shows itself to be otherwise than what first appears. Specifically I reflected on and described the weakness of my power. When confronted by the gaze of another, this vulnerable Other reveals to me that my own power has a tendency toward violence and therefore reveals the very source of my weakness as fault. I *am exposed.* I am turned inside out. Trying to *expose* the Other, I find my own weakness *exposed.* Furthermore, I find her power and weakness beyond my comprehension, control, and consumption. I *confess* my violence, which is exposed by the Other. I am commanded to say, "Here I am. I am guilty."

In chapter 6, I began to attend to the other side of the paradox, namely, that the face of the Other not only justly accuses me of the weakness of power, but also calls me to go beyond my guilt and to be ethically responsible to and for the neediness of the Other. The phenomenological method for reflecting and describing was to *listen to and be touched by* this call to be ethical, and to *respond,* "Here I am. I am responsible to listen to, to serve, to have patience and compassion and to celebrate with the Other." This was a *phenomenology of responsibility.*

So far I have described two kinds of *individualism: egological individualism,* where the self assumes its center to be in itself, calculates, and manipulates ways to keep that center, and a *psukhological individualism,* where the self is breathed into me by the neediness and dignity of the Other. This latter is what Levinas calls "ethical individualism," or "responsible individualism." The "I," knowing it is responsible, must ask itself, "How am I, as an individual, responsible to the individual Other?"

Finally, I recognize another *responsible individualism*, as *community individualism*. Adopting a psukhology that would be the study of responsibility breathed not only into the psukhe of the "I," and from the psukhe of the "I" breathing responsibility into the Other, but also into other Others, into all Others, into the community, I must ask, "How am I, as an member of community, responsible to other Others through social institutions and their structures?" Here, in chapter 7, I begin a *phenomenology of community*. My experience in community reveals that I am connected and responsible not only to the immediate Other, but also to all others. I am called by all others.

COMMUNITIES UNDERSTOOD BY USING THE THREE LEVELS OF THE PSUKHE: COGNITION, BEHAVIOR, AFFECT

This call by multiple others commands me to *reason* about another paradox: *Because I am called to responsibility, I must limit my responding.* The limitations placed on altruism because of the existence of other Others, discussed in the Interlude, calls me to compare incomparables. This requirement to *compare incomparables* is the basis for *understanding with reason:* I must try to *figure things out* and make good judgments and right choices about others who are each ethically worthy. I must reflect not only on my responsibility, but also on the responsibility of others to other Others. I must engage in conversation and action with others to design, organize, and implement how each person's responsibility fits into the complex of responsibilities, and how we all fit together not simply to provide for the common good as the whole, but for the common good to serve the good of each individual.

Since not only is there never just one other person *to whom* I am responsible, but also others *with whom* I am responsible, I must incorporate my personal responsibility and work within a reasoning and responsible community working for the common good. Since I cannot figure things out by myself, cannot reason to every proper conclusion, I must join others in *community reasoning*. The phenomenological method for a community's reflecting on and describing this paradox of each person's answering to her or his responsibility, checking the limits to her or his own response, and calculating each other person's responsibility, is to reason with others in the community setting through *public discourse*. Reason is not the human faculty that first and foremost defines the condition of being an individual human. Rather, reason grows out of shared community responsibility. Responsibility as the condition of the human has ontological priority over reason as an individual event. *Reason* serves *responsibility*. Responsibility does not develop out of reason.

Since each person is responsible for all yet cannot do it all, we need to design and reasonably use the institutions of society. The principle institution for reasoning and teaching about the distribution of rights and responsibility and the skills to carry these out is the *educational community*. Educational activity is certainly not confined to the places called *schools*. Any institutional public conversation to learn about and articulate our shared responsibility is an academic community. Schools, however, have a special obligation to carry this out with disinterested interest. Academia is the community exercising its ethical power at the *cognitive* level of *knowing*. Cynicism grows when the members of the community watch academia pursue self-interest.

Besides rational discourse in the academic community, we must each *commit* to cooperative and competitive action with each other to actually assure rights and responsibilities, for social justice for all. The principle institution for determining and assuring rights and responsibilities is the *political community*. Political activity is certainly not confined to the places called *government*. Any public institution established by the citizens to fulfill their responsibility through just means is a political community. Governments, however, have a special obligation to carry this out with disinterested interest. Politics is the way the community exercises, at the *behavioral* level of *acting*, its ethical power to guarantee justice for all. Cynicism grows when the members of the community watch politicians pursue self-interest.

Besides the academic community, which is the social structure for reasoning toward the good of each person and the common good, and the political community, which is for carrying out justice for individuals and for the society as a whole, each of us is called to show compassion for those marginalized from the academic and political communities. Compassion must be shown in providing for the needs of everyone. The principle institution for providing for others through the just distribution of goods and services is the *commercial community*. Commercial activity is certainly not confined to the places called *businesses*. Any public institution established to compassionately exchange goods and services is an economic community. Businesses, however, have a special obligation to carry this out with disinterested interest. Economics is the way the community exercises at the affective level of feeling its ethical power to provide the material needs of all citizens. Cynicism grows when the members of the community watch businesses solely pursue self-interest.

Etymologically, the word *economics* comes from the Greek *oikonomia* (*oikos* "house" + *nemein* "to manage"). To the extent that economics has evolved into competition for individual self-interest and neglected the compassionate interest of the Other in the house, for all in the house, all in the community, all humanity, it is violence. This does not mean that the best means for justly distributing goods and services for everyone in the community could not be a system with competition. Certainly, we have seen the inherent destructiveness of a system that eliminates competition and centrally plans its economic activity. But a system that supports individual responsibility for planning economic activity ought to keep as its first principle (actually its first fact) that every individual is responsible for the good of every other and for the common good through responsibility to and for the Other. Responsibility to the self follows responsibility to the Other.

Community responsibility to individual others by individual others and to the community as a whole ought to include justice for "even the undeserving," as Bishop Untener (1991) urges us. Requirements for social justice ought to support the inherent, ethical rights of everyone, regardless of the level of their contribution as educational, political, and commercial participants. Fundamental rights are based on the infinite goodness of each person, not on what they *deserve* calculated according to their intellectual, productive, or financial contribution. If rights to *get* were based only on what the person *gives*, then there would be no *rights*, only *return payments* or *rewards*. The giving/getting model describes nature's laws. Pure reciprocal giving and getting does not define an ethical humanity. We all suffer under this narrow system modeled after Newtonian laws of action and reaction. One of Dorothy Day's often repeated quips was, "God help us all if we got just what we deserved."

It seems to me that there are three fundamental social injustices that call us to organize our educational, political, and commercial communities and to act responsibly through them. These issues are based not on any calculus of reciprocal contribution, but on an ethics of deserving through the inherent worthiness of the recipients of justice. These are social causes par excellence:

1. Guaranteeing the respect and rights of marginalized individuals and groups: racial, ethnic, gender, age, disabled, sexual orientation. People in economic classes who suffer disabling poverty in our contemporary vicious market system especially call us to community responsibility.
2. Protecting and educating children who are the communities of the future.
3. Saving the precious earth not only because from it we all receive the goods for our lives, but also because of its inherent dignity.

I will describe an understanding of the social institutions designed in their own way to address these social causes par excellence.

Educational Community

The face of the Other calls me to *simplicity*, to be skeptical of my judgments about the Other and to be open to her teaching me about herself. As a member of a community, I am called to know as much as I can about the needs of others, both as individuals and as a community. My primary source of knowledge of others is in the face-to-face meeting. But I am also called to understand those others who are beyond face-to-face opportunities. An open and democratic society organized by and for the people rests solidly on its citizens' being informed and thoughtful about others. Each member ought to be perceptive of injustice and rational in their deliberations about ways to reform persons and society. For the citizens to be well informed and thoughtful in the use of democratic structures, the society must have good schools, a responsible media, and organized and spontaneous street-level forums for discussing the issues. I am called to participate in these institutions and structures. If I am to be a responsible member of the community, I must seek to be educated and confident in the knowledge I have gained.

While the face of the Other calls me to simplicity, to self-skepticism about my judgments of others, I too easily use the excuse of my ignorance about others to release myself from community responsibilities. My claim that I do not know about the needs of others is often an indication that I have no interest in the needs of others. An interest in their needs does not serve my self-interest. Mediocrity is the secret of my contentment.

Against my tendency toward this selfishness, I am called to be skeptical about my excuse of ignorance, which is secretly based on my lack of interest in others. The face of the Other calls me to be interested in her needs and in the needs of the community over and above my self-interest. I am called to learn about community issues through discourse with other members in order to make judgments and choices for the good of the community that serve the good of its individual members. Naiveté is not an acceptable excuse to avoid discourse. We are educated within discourse with others. Community members are called to turn their ignorance into that kind of simplicity that is open to each other in listening to each other's needs. I have the ethical responsibility to learn from others and to call other Others to community responsibility.

A community is called to a *collective simplicity* in order to gain disinterested knowledge about each other. Disinterested knowledge is knowledge about the good of the community independent of individual self-interest. As a society raises its level of complexity of knowledge, it becomes more difficult for every citizens to understand its structures and processes. This brings about an uneven distribution of knowledge. Our arrogance about the knowledge we possess tends to urge us to judge, through that narrow perspective, the intentions of others. We lapse into ideological divisiveness and cynicism. When citizens are confronted with what they judge to be too much information about issues and candidates, they tend to seek "simplicity" by clinging to ideological certainties, answers that serve only their own best interest. These ideological certainties reduce others to stereotypes that distort the truth about others. These distorted certainties tend to be *simplistic* without being *simple* in the sense of being open to the other. *Ideological simplicity,* reduction of others to stereotypes and exclusion from them, is the counterforce of the *collective simplicity* that urges us to be open to each other through community discourse. Ideologies divide people into competing viewpoints and urge each faction to be cynical about those who do not share their certainties. While there will always be differences between viewpoints on community issues, seductive ideologies that urge deep divisiveness and cynicism can undermine the fundamental responsibility every member has toward every other member.

We are all somewhat naive when it comes to knowing each other. We have the obligation to be open to learn from each other and remain in a kind of wonder. The word *naive* comes from the Latin *nasci,* to be born. We are all young. We are new to each other even though we have known each other for a long time. The otherness of the Other makes each moment of meeting as if for the first time. What a joy. While schools train individuals in skills, their primary responsibility is to develop community by inspiring responsibility.

Political Community

The face of the Other calls me to *humility,* to substitute myself in the service of the Other and of all other Others. As a member of the community I am called to actively contribute to the good of others by involving myself in the political structures and processes of the various levels of government that allow me to extend my reach to those beyond my immediate reach. All those others must have universal access to the protections and benefits of the governments to provide me the means to serve those others.

Governments should not only provide the structures and processes to invest in its citizens the freedom to act responsibly toward others, they should also inspire a *collective humility,* one that urges all citizens to fulfill their responsibility by collectively serving others by means of social institutions.

Governments have two problems. First of all, the large organization of government tends to take the broad perspective and overlook the needs of individuals and to reduce them to the stereotypes of its broad categories. The bureaucratic processes of governments, in their effort to become efficient on a large scale, tend to become compulsively routine. Governing should be democratic, not only by giving universal access to its benefits, but also by allowing citizens to easily watch its particular behavior and to correct its abuses when it violates the rights of individuals. Open and frequent voting must guard against abuse. Open, fair, and frequent elections are *permanent revolutions.*

Governments require permanent revolutions to guard against intermittent chaotic and violent revolutions that inevitably arise to overthrow oppressive regimes. Permanent revolutions must always be sensitive to the suffering of the most vulnerable members of the community. It is so often said that the character of a society can be judged by the way it treats its poor.

Paradoxically, the call for permanent revolution, while inherently *progressive*, is also the call to be *conservative*, to hold on to traditions until they have clearly proven themselves to be harmful, and to be cautious of unproven innovations that could bring even greater injustice. Without permanent revolution, simultaneously progressive and conservative, societies calcify into paranoid protectionism and suspicion, righteousness based on ignorance, inert habits, and greed, rather than justice.

The second problem of governments is the tendency of individuals, driven by compulsive self-interest, to "use the system" of governments, not as the means to serve others, but as the means to gain special privileges for themselves and their social and ideological groups. Large and complicated systems are susceptible to manipulation by clever operators. It is cynically accepted by too many people to "use the system" of big government for self-interested gain rather than to use government as the means to substitute one's own service for others.

Celebrations of the community's inspirational origins and successes are necessary to preserve the enjoyment of individual goods within the common good. Celebrations appear through customary ceremonies such as the rites of passage of the young, the inauguration of authority, and festivals that re-member (*re-* "again" + *-memo* "be mindful") the community's struggles and successes. Celebrations reassemble the values upon which the community came together. Celebrations shake us from our tendency toward self-interested individualism and inspire us to fulfill our responsibility to others and to the community.

Disinterested effort in work for others requires *collective humility*, in which we labor for each other and the common good. As a society raises its level of social control by the use of mechanical and bureaucratic technologies, it must guard against the violence of anonymous systems that generalize individuals into statistics and disregard their individual rights and responsibilities, and it must guard against the manipulation of its complex systems by individuals who are taking advantage of "the system."

Commercial Community

The face of the Other calls me to *patience*, sacrificing my enjoyment so that the needs of the Other and of all other Others can be fulfilled. As a member of the community, I am called to generously provide goods for the needs of others, even those beyond my own helping hand. To provide for others, there must be an economic system that guarantees justice in the distribution of the goods and services to all members of the community.

At the heart of distributive justice is gratitude. Robert Louis Stevenson's lines, "The world is so full of a number of things, I'm sure we should all be as happy as kings" (1950) should be a mantra for the citizens of contemporary society. Enjoyment is not a lapse of seriousness, but the love of life. I contribute to the community by enjoying goods. If I sacrifice enjoyment because I judge goods to be evil or false, out of some ascetic philosophy, my giving of these goods would be contributing to the harm of others. I sacrifice for others not because things are bad for me, but because things are good for me and for the Other who has rights to them over me.

Just as compassion for one's neighbor requires gratitude for what one has been given, so greediness is built on envy for what one has not. This greediness is the flaw of our present marketing system, so dependent on advertising, that convinces us that we are unhappy because of something we have not got. Most advertising has become *psychogogy* (*psukhe* "soul" + *agein* "to lead"). It seduces our psyches into believing that we need beyond our needs. Modern advertising urges us to be envious of the characters in the advertisement who have what we do not have. Just as envy is used to inspire greed, so gratitude for the gratuitousness of gifts provides the basis to give to those who suffer. Our patience is suffering for the sake of the others because they have rights over us to fill their needs and we have gratitude for what we have.

As a member of the community, I must not only contribute goods to other members of the community, but I must also work to urge others to share responsibly. Although the *ideal* notion of "all receiving according to their needs" is a Marxist utopia that can never be achieved, we must, however, have a "preferential option for the poor" articulated so forcefully by the Latin American bishops at their Medellin Conference of 1968. In an economy of *free enterprise*, the weakest in the community tend to suffer.

Therefore, we should ethically prefer the poor in order to guard against the abuse of the economically weakest. The psychogogy of advertising seduces consumers to thoughtlessly indulge. If the affluent indulge thoughtlessly and develop gripping addictions, their psyches can be corrupted into an ignorance of their responsibility. While the poor and uneducated are often the most helpless pawns of the media and advertising, when the poor are freed from thoughtless indulgence, they have a clearer understanding of their situation, and of the need to share more responsibly.

As a society increases the production and distribution of consumer goods, it must guard against extreme concentrations of wealth and poverty, the addiction of its consumers, and destruction of the environment. Decency and fairness should call us to *collective patience, gratitude and compassion.*

THE POWER OF THE COMMON GOOD IN SCHOOLS , GOVERNMENTS, AND BUSINESSES

My question to myself is, how am I to be responsible for others by contributing to the common good of the community, a contribution that in turn extends my responsibility for other individuals within the community? I will follow the outline used in chapters 3, 4, 5, and 6 for the five modes of interpersonal relationships: self-centering, serving others, cooperating, competing, exercising leadership. Each of these are described on the cognitive, behavioral, and affective levels of the psyche.

Self-Centering for the Common Good

Everyone has the obligation to the common good to offer themselves as talented and experienced. I am responsible to develop my talents not only in order to carry out my individual task, but also to join in the overall tasks of the society. These talents are developed not only in formal schooling, but also from all information resources and training programs such as libraries, media, and especially social conversations in families, neighborhoods, friendships, workplace alliances, professional organizations, even in small talk on the street. To contribute oneself to the community, one must have knowledge and skill to offer a worthy contribution.

COMPARING ONESELF IN THE GROUP TO UNDERSTAND INDIVIDUAL ROLE

Although the Other always takes ethical precedence over the self, the self must compare his talents and situation to others in order to judge what contributions must be made. Certainly, our society has at times placed too much emphasis on comparing the self with others. Students get discouraged because of comparisons in school. They may overlook their own natural talents, developed skills, and preferred rewards when they attend too much to the success of others. However, there can be too much of the contrary effort to encourage students to *do your own thing*. Community success requires that individuals self-reflect and find their place in the group. This requires comparisons with others.

DISCIPLINING ONESELF TO THE GROUP STANDARDS TO IMPROVE SKILLS
FOR THE COMMON GOOD

The self must discipline itself, to be a *disciple* of the community. Although the word "disciple" has evolved into some negative connotations, like "member of a cult," it comes from the Latin word *discipulus*, pupil or student, from *discere* to learn. To discipline oneself means to develop knowledge and skills so that the self can contribute to the established good of the community. Certainly, the standards of groups can be oppressive and retard the imagination and autonomy of individuals. But group customs serve the purpose of guiding choices as to what is acceptable and what might be judged as inappropriate. Knowing the customs is essential in order to deviate and set up uniquely new community actions. Everyone needs to feel welcomed in a community. Knowing how the other members of the community act improves the chances of this welcome.

FASTING FOR SELF-NOURISHING AND TO EXPERIENCE SOLIDARITY
IN THE SUFFERING OF OTHERS

The self must sacrifice its consumption of goods, not just to share those goods with others, but also to condition his/her own physiological and psychological health in order to contribute to the good of the community. The word *diet* comes from the Greek *diaita*, meaning "a way of living." Although, most frequently, we use the word *diet* to mean fasting from certain foods and including other foods, we also use the term to refer to any careful exclusion and inclusion of goods in our daily habits of consuming.

Serving Others for the Common Good

I can contribute not only to the needs of specific others by serving goods to them, but also I can serve the common good of the community, which can serve still other Others. Parents' care for their children, children's care for their elderly parents, neighbors' care for neighbors, all reduce the cost to the community as a whole. Those served children, parents and neighbors, can then further contribute to the common good of the community.

The viewpoint of the weakest members of society is the most difficult to understand. Their viewpoint is hidden because they have less power to express it to others. Powerful others often avoid the viewpoint of weak members because the experience is uncomfortable and often painful. Even when the appeal of the weak is heard, it carries little power on its own. The viewpoint of the weak has power only when it calls into question the self-interested viewpoint of the powerful. When powerful members see the truth of the suffering of others, this truth can have the power to call these powerful persons to question the injustices that have been brought about by the weakening of others. Truth ought to be sought for the sake of knowing reality. The perspective of the weak has no value other than the truth of reality.

It might be objected that the weak often take advantage of others and distort the truth for their own interest. They cheat, lie, steal, and even kill. When they act out of pure self-interest, their motives are not from the conditions for truth gotten from suffering weakness. Their motives are from the position of those seeking power, perhaps even by using their weakness as a manipulative lever against others. The viewpoint of the weak is the experience of the raw reality of the necessities of life, unbuffered by the luxuries and conveniences of those who are not weak. The needs and conditions of life are starkest from the viewpoint of the weak.

Everyone knows this naked truth when they have found themselves in positions of weakness. We have sympathy for others from comparing our experiences with theirs. The problem with sympathy is that we tend to reduce the Other's weakness to one equivalent to our own. This reduction distorts the truth of the Other. Empathy, however, involves feeling for the Other's suffering by comparing our suffering with the Other's, yet respects the absolute otherness, the uniqueness of the Other. The viewpoint of the weakest members of society can give us an understanding of reality closest to the truth when we honor the dignity of their absolute otherness.

At the cognitive level, we serve the common good by knowing that the otherness of others is beyond our fully knowing because they have infinite dignity as humans, and thus are worthy of honor as Other. When we judge others by reducing them to the list of faults they have committed or selfishness they have displayed, then we have reduced ourselves as ignorant. Judging others is not authentic simplicity. It is not open to the infinite otherness of others beyond our understanding.

The first good effect of volunteering is to alleviate some of the suffering of others. The common good is improved when fewer suffer. The logic of this seems all too obvious.

The second good effect of volunteering is to better understand the systemic problems of an unjust society in order to work with other members of the community to change the system. That is why volunteers should do more than relieve suffering. They should publicly express concern and contribute some way to bring about structural change for permanent revolutions.

PROVIDING CHARITABLE AND COMMERCIAL GOODS

It certainly makes sense for smaller independent institutions to handle what they can without demanding that larger public ones take over. Families, neighborhoods, workplace groups, friendships, and groups organized around common interests can help their own members before turning to larger bureaucracy for help. Citizens, however, should try to understand the complexity of the issues before they resist contributing money to the common good by way of taxes and other charity. The paradox of power and weakness can help us get a deeper understanding of the role of taxes and government funding of the weak and marginalized in our society.

Cooperating in the Community for the Common Good

Each member of the community has an obligation to cooperate with others to bring about the *permanent revolution*, consistent watchfulness and change. Citizenship must be defined more by the responsibilities owed to the community than by the rights each expects to receive. When we depend only on others to fill community obligations, we are committing injustice against those others.

BECOMING INFORMED

Patriotism and other forms of supporting institutional structures are important. Essential to the *moral voice* of a community are defenders of the system. This does not mean we should be loyal to a power faction that oppresses other groups. It means that authorities need to hear from people who are well served by their structure as well as hear from those who have complaints. Voicing criticism against the unjust structures abusing others, especially the weakest members of society, is an essential form of patriotism. Patriotism is defending the common good by defending the rights of individuals protected by the government.

PARTICIPATING IN COMMUNITY ACTION

Besides voting, there are other formal means of organizing, advocating, and politicking, such as serving on school boards, health boards, neighborhood councils, other advisory commissions, juries, and many more. There are informal means such as letter writing, telephone and door-to-door canvasing, leaflet distributing, and other activities that seek political changes. These activities can take place within government structures, local and national, or they can be in public but nongovernment locations such as the workplace, labor unions, schools, professional associations, churches, and so forth.

Often staunch defenders of the party in power criticize those who get involved in political activism that protests government. The defenders of government may be motivated to avoid conflict, or they may place too much trust in governing officials. Democracies require that citizens watch those in power to assure they enhance the common good, which can then provide for each individual good.

SUPPORTING AND BOYCOTTING BUSINESSES

Perhaps the first form of supporting the economic system is paying taxes. There are certainly unjust tax systems that we are obliged to protest and legally undo. But paying money to governments to provide goods and services to the less fortunate beyond our individual reach and to provide public facilities available to everyone is fundamental to the community well-being.

The major form of supporting the economy is to work for an income and spend those wages for needed goods. The competitive market where prices are kept in check by others challenging with lower prices can only work if a reasonably large number of customers shop. However, just as dieting by controlling one's own consumption of goods is good for the individual, so does it contribute to the common good. The major reason to limit our consuming is to preserve the environment. Our ecological problems are directly linked to our consumer-oriented economy. If we continue to ingest our natural resources and pile up waste at the present rate, we will destroy the earth for everyone. The most vicious consequence of our environmental degradation is that the first victims of our present abuse are the poor who cannot protect themselves from pollution, and the second victims will be the descendants of everyone. They will have no escape from the poverty of our greedy depletion and the pollutants of our arrogant negligence.

Competing in the Community by Challenging Others for the Common Good

Not only is cooperation good, but so is competition between political parties, as well as between other groups with vested interests, when that competition is a challenge that serves the challenged rather than an attack to reduce the competitor.

PUBLICLY QUESTIONING THE SOCIAL STRUCTURES

Debating public policy and practices is essentially competing with alternative understandings in order to arrive at the truth. We ought to be able to have trust in the very process of open debate rather than in the use of seductive or coercive methods to get people to support ideologies that serve the vested interests of exclusive groups. Criticizing the operation of public institutions is an important contribution to this public debate.

Certainly each person is called differently in this obligation to criticize parts of society. Some are called to discuss issues with family and neighbors, some to attend public forums, some to stand up and speak out at these forums, some to write letters to officials and to the media. Some more formally write and speak as recognized social critics and some become opposition candidates for political offices and agency directors.

Too frequently people read and discuss politics selectively. They tend to only read biased pieces and dialogue with whom they already agree. Most cynical carping takes place behind walls that keep the criticism from reaching the ears of those who should hear and could make changes.

CHALLENGING THE POLICIES AND PRACTICES OF POWER STRUCTURES

When we challenge those who have power, we make them sharpen their sense of ethics and their skills in achieving the good. These challenges should be motivated out of a real concern for arriving at not only the most efficient structures and practices, but also for the most humane.

INVESTING IN SOCIALLY RESPONSIBLE BUSINESSES

Searching for the best quality and the most competitive prices can contribute to the common good. But alone it pushes the weak to the margins of society. When those who can afford their cost boycott products because it is unjust for those who cannot afford them, those more affluent ones contribute to the common good. When affordable products become less available because their sellers cannot stay in business, then the affluent have some obligation either to buy lower-priced products in order to keep them available, or to influence the market forces in other ways to keep affordable goods available to the poor.

Exercising Leadership by Participative Management

Leaders have a special obligation to contribute to the common good by providing for the good of those individuals over whom they have authority. With the power of the subordinates invested in the leaders, those leaders have the opportunity to articulate the reasons for the common good, putting into effect practices that serve the common good and justly distributing the benefits of the common good.

ARTICULATING THE COMMUNITY'S VISION AND NEEDS

The task of the leader is to balance four elements: (1) to produce a quality service or product; (2) to assure good morale in the work-place; (3) to gain a profit for the owners; and (4) to commit to use the organization as a vehicle for positive social change. To give these elements due effort, the leader must calculate the importance of each, plan how to manage employees and resources, and evaluate the balance of these for further management. The last element (social consciousness) may be considered least by many organizations, especially for-profit businesses. However, business theorists not only articulate the ethical command to contribute to the common good for the sake of the common good, they also show how it increases profit, raises morale among employees, and therefore raises productivity, especially in the form of the improvement of the quality of the service or product.

IMPLEMENTING THE COMMUNITY'S PROGRAMS

Management techniques to fulfill the four elements of a good organization are becoming more and more sophisticated. I cannot presume to describe these, but will trust in the articulation of those who are in leadership roles and those who intellectually attend to these practices.

DEVELOPING SOCIAL GROWTH, NOT NECESSARILY ECONOMIC GROWTH

Leaders of both public and private organizations and institutions must focus on growth. This focus may not mean economic growth if that development will bring damage to the environment and suffering to some sectors of society, especially the poor. The overall quality of the lifestyle of all members of the community is essential. Although businesses may be in competition for producing and selling, they can work together to provide a satisfied and compassionate community. Organizations are called to measure the unmeasurables, those inside and outside the organization. The preferential option for the poor is simply the demand to put special effort into assuring their economic rights. When the economic forces of the market are left to themselves they can bring unjust hardships to those who do not have the knowledge, the skills, and the capital to provide for themselves. Therefore, businesses have a special obligation to support the poor.

CONCLUSION

The philosophy of radical altruism that finds each individual responsible for others should be at the center of the social philosophy that guides educational, political, and economic policies and practices. Although I have tended to focus in the earlier chapters on the psychological view of existence, this last chapter has attempted to articulate the sociological view. My lack of sophistication in theory and practice in social, political, and economic structures and processes is evident. I have made this effort in order to urge others with greater knowledge and skill in these areas, perhaps motivated by my naiveté, to take up the issues I have briefly touched upon.

Epilogue

When I visited Dr. Levinas in his home in Paris, he wrote inside the cover of my copy of his *Collected Philosophical Papers* the following line: *Avec tous mes regrets devant une occasion de sympathie active—manquée, Paris le 2 juin 87*,[1] and then his scribbled signature.

I could not translate all of his message, especially the last word, *manquée*. Back home, a French teacher told me that although literally it means *"lack,"* he probably meant *"missed opportunity."* During our visit I had understood very little of Levinas's French and he had understood more but not all of my English. Our conversation dealt mostly with being on holiday in France, our children's names, that we had come from Seattle, that it was kind of him to give us a few minutes. I fumbled around trying to express my gratitude for his philosophy and why and how I taught it to graduate students in a therapeutic psychology program. He made it clear enough that he had difficulty understanding how his philosophy could be of any use to psychologists. I had first understood that the message he wrote expressing *regrets* for *une occasion manquée* referred only to our somewhat uncomfortable thirty-minute visit. But as I have come to know his philosophy better over these few years I have taken the liberty to interpret his 1987 note to have a wider meaning.

We are incessantly haunted by feelings of *regret* that we "have not done enough" and that, although the future is *the-time-we-have-left*, the past holds memories of *opportunities missed*. For example, I did not express enough gratitude to my parents before they died, both suddenly without my presence. When I later heard of Dr. Levinas's illness, I had planned to write him once more, but I regret that I did not get around to it. A list of my regrets could be endless and boring.

---

1. I have left this inscription and other names in the epilogue in the original French rather than their translation out of respect for Levinas's original words.

Levinas's philosophy teaches me how to understand why I never fully meet my responsibilities. It is not only that my intelligence, effort, and compassion fall short because of my tendency toward selfishness, but the Other is also *always-more-than* I could ever understand, ever fill her or his needs, and ever adequately feel compassion for. I am always called and always unable to reach the absolute otherness of the Other and always responsible to do more. Rather than defining the future as *on-the-way-toward-death*, Levinas tells us that the future is *the-time-we-have-left*. He writes, "To be conscious is to have time" (1961/69, p. 237). Regrets can be partly redeemed.

Levinas's philosophy of time attends not only to *regret*, but also to *forgiveness* and *hope*:

> The will, already betrayal and alienation of itself but postponing this betrayal, on the way to death but a death ever future, exposed to death but not *immediately*, has time to be for the Other, and thus to recover meaning despite death. (1961/69, p. 236)

Human existence, for Levinas, is *being-responsible-for-the-Other-before-death*.

Only now, after Levinas died on December 25, 1995, do many of us, outside elite circles of Continental philosophers, Jewish theologians, and a few literary scholars, seriously pick up his work. Attention to him was a long time coming. When he was twenty-four in 1930, he introduced phenomenology to France, with his dissertation, *"Théorie de l'intuition dans la phénoménologie de Husserl."* The following year he co-translated an expanded version of the lectures Husserl gave in Paris in February 1920, entitled Cartesian Meditations (1931). Levinas authored numerous articles on phenomenology from the late 1920s to the early 1980s. He was silenced when captured as a French military officer, and he spent time at forced labor in a prison camp. His parents and brothers were murdered in Eastern Europe by collaborators of the German Nazis. Much of the time before and after the war he modestly taught at the École Israélite Orientale du Bassin Méditerranéen. Only in 1961 did Levinas gain much notice by publishing his main thesis for the *doctorat d'État: Totalité et infini*, and more when he published *Autrement qu'être ou au-delà de l'essence*, in 1974.

Although we psychologists can regret the missed opportunity of his life that we did not discover the value of his philosophy while he was alive, we can be *in-the-time-before-death* of psychology. We can benefit from his challenge to *egology* and, inspired by his philosophy of *responsibility*, take notice of the psychological experiences of responsible graciousness that blesses the lives of many and is too frequently absent from the lives of many of those we know and serve. Psychology, trying to liberate itself from philosophical, theological, and other cultural "myths," and trying to liberate individuals from the oppression of others, as well it should, has too often only provided alternative self-sabotaging seductions and illusions of egocentrism. A psychology of *radical altruism* can reveal these seductions and illusions and the universal call to responsibility.

There is another simple notion that helps summarize the philosophy of Emmanuel Levinas. Sander Goodheart told me that when visiting with Levinas in that same apartment in Paris a few years before his death, Levinas said that it all comes down to *la politesse*, to politeness or kindness. Levinas continued with Sander on the theme that the politeness that provides the context within which we can carry on our daily activity is often trivialized. I assume, knowing his concerns about modern philosophy and social sciences, he meant that scholars trivialize *la politesse* in their analysis. My reading of Levinas has inspired me to recognize that psychologists have overlooked this fundamental social "ether" of *la politesse* that we inhale and exhale and that nourishes the sinews and bones of our psyches.

Although I do not expect, or even desire, the term *psukhology* to catch on, I hope psychology can recognize and study not only the *possibilities* of radical altruism, but also its *commonness* and its *power* to heal. Psychology has staked out its subject matter based on the cynical assumption of *self-interest*. But, for the most part, people do not act toward one another out of self-interest. In his interview with Philippe Nemo (1982/85), Levinas had just defined the *self* with the statement, "I am he who finds the resources to respond to the call."

Nemo retorted, "One is tempted to say to you: yes, in some cases. But in other cases, to the contrary, the encounter with the Other occurs in the mode of violence, hate and disdain."

Levinas's response:

> To be sure. But I think that whatever the motivation which explains this inversion, the analysis of the face such as I have just made, with the mastery of the Other and his poverty, and my submission and my wealth, is primary. It is the presupposed in all human relationships. If it were not that, we would not even say, before an open door, "After you, sir!" It is an original "After you, sir!" that I have tried to describe. (1982/85, p. 89)

I would like to call this epilogue a second prologue because I hope it will be a beginning. Psychology now has available to it a foundational philosophy of *responsibility* in the wisdom revealed by Emmanuel Levinas.

Bibliography

Bellah, Robert, R. Mudson, W. Sullivan, A. Swidler, and S. Tipton. (1985). *Habits of the Heart*. Berkeley: University of California Press.

Batson, C. D. (1991). *The Altruism Question: Toward a Social-psychological Answer*. Hillsdale, NJ: Erlbaum.

Burggraeve, Roger. (1985). *From Self-Development to Solidarity: An Ethical Reading of Human Desire in Its Socio-Political Relevance according to Emmanuel Levinas*. (C. Vanhove-Romanik, Trans.). Leuven, Belgium: Peeters Publishers.

Burke, John Patrick. (1982). "The Ethical Significance of the Face." Paper read at the Fifty-sixth Annual Meeting of the American Catholic Philosophical Association, Houston, Texas. Camus, Albert. (1847/1948). *The Plague*. (Stuart Gilbert, Trans.) New York: Random House.

Cialdini, R. B., M. Schaller, D. Houlihan, K. Arps, J. Fultz, and A. L. Beamen, (1987). "Empathy-Based helping: Is It Selflessly or Selfishly Motivated?" *Journal of Personality and Social Psychology* 52: 749–58.

Cushman, Philip. (1990). "Why the Self Is Empty: Toward a Historically Situated Psychology." *American Psychologist* 45. 5, 599–611.

Daly, Markate. (1994). *Communitarianism: A New Public Ethics*. Belmont, CA: Wadsworth.

de Boer, Theo. (1983). *Foundations of a Critical Psychology* (Theodore Plantinga, Trans.) Pittsburgh: Duquesne University Press.

Derrida, Jacques. (1964/1978). "Violence and Metaphysics." In *Writing and Difference* (Alan Bass, Trans.). Chicago: Chicago University Press.

Dickinson, Emily. (1958). *The Poems of Emily Dickinson*. (Thomas H. Johnson, Ed.) Cambridge, MA: The Belknap Press.

Dovidio, J. F., J. Allen, and S. A. Schroeder. (1990). "The Specificity of Empathy-Induced Helping: Evidence for Altruism." *Journal of Personality and Social Psychology* 59: 249–60.

Dostoyevsky, Fyodor. (1957) *The Brothers Karamazov* (Constance Garnett, Trans.). New York: New American Library.

Etizoni, Amitai. (1988). *The Moral Dimension: Toward a New Economics.* New York: Free Press.

———, 1990–94. ed. *The Responsive Community.* 4 vols.

———. (1993). *The Spirit of Community: Rights, Responsibilities, and The Communitarian Agenda.* New York: Crown.

Giorgi, Amedeo. (1970). *Psychology as a Human Science.* New York: Harper & Row.

Grant, M. & Hazel, John. (1973). *Gods and Mortals in Classical Mythology.* Springfield, MA: Merriam-Webster.

Greenberg, Gary. (1994). *The Self on the Shelf: Recovery Books and the Good Life.* Albany: State University of New York Press.

Greene, Graham. (1961). *The Burnt-out Case.* New York: Viking Press.

———, (1970). *The Power and the Glory.* New York: Viking Press.

Greenleaf, Robert. (1977). *Servant Leadership: A Journey into the Nature of Legitimate Power and Greatness.* New York: Paulist Press.

Habermas, Jürgen. (1972). *Knowledge and Human Interest.* Boston: Beacon Press.

Halling, Steen. (1975). "The Implications of Emmanuel Levinas' *Totality and Infinity* for Therapy." In *Duquesne Studies in Phenomenological Psychology: Volume II* (Amedeo Giorgi, Constance T. Fischer, and Edward L. Murray, Eds.). Pittsburgh: Duquesne University Press.

Halling, Steen, Georg Kunz, and Jan Rowe. (1994). "The Contributions of Dialogal Psychology to Phenomenological Research." *Journal of Humanistic Psychology* 34. 1 pp. 109–131.

Halling, S., M. Leifer, C. Menuhin-Hauser, K. Pape, and J. O. Rowe. (1992, June). "When Injustice Cannot be Ignored: Living as Social Activists." Paper presented at the 11th International Human Science Research Conference, Oakland University, Rochester, MI.

Hatley, James. (1996). "Prophetic Subjectivity: Inwardness without Secrets." Paper read at the Society for Existential-Phenomenological Philosophy Conference, Chicago.

Heidegger, Martin. (1962). *Being and Time* (John Macquarrie and Edward Robinson, Trans.). New York: Harper & Row. (Original work published in 1927)

Husserl, Edmund. (1913/1962). *Ideas: General Introduction to Pure Phenomenology* (W. R. Gibson, Trans.). New York: Collier.

———. (1931/1960). *Cartesian Meditations.* (Dorion Cairns, Trans.). The Hague: Martinus Nijhoff.

Kohn, Alfie, (1986). *No Contest: The Case against Competition.* Boston: Houghton Mifflin.

Leddy, Mary Jo. (1991). "Formation in a Post-Modern Context." *Way Supplement*, 71: 6–15.

Levinas, Emmanuel. (1961/1969). *Totality and Infinity* (Alfonso Lingis, Trans.). Pittsburgh: Duquesne University Press.

———. (1973). *The Theory of Intuition in Husserl's Phenomenology* (Andre Orianne, Trans.). Evanston, IL: Northwestern University Press. (Original work published in 1963)

———. (1974/1981). *Otherwise Than Being or Beyond Essence.* (Alfonso Lingis, Trans.). The Hague: Martinus Nijhoff.

———. (1978). *Existence and Existents* (Alfonso Lingis, Trans.). The Hague: Martinus Nijhoff.

———. (1982/1985). *Ethics and Infinity* (Richard Cohen, Trans.). Pittsburgh: Duquesne University Press.

———. (1988). "Useless Suffering." In *The Provocation of Levinas,* edited by Robert Bernasconi and David Wood. London: Routledge, pp. 156–67.

Manning, Robert John Sheffler. (1993). *Interpreting Otherwise than Heidegger.* Pittsburgh: Duquesne University Press.

Menzies, Heather. (1996). *Whose Brave New World? The Information Highway and the New Economy.* Toronto: Between the Lines Publishing Company.

MacIntyre, Alasdair. (1981). *After Virtue.* Notre Dame, Indiana: University of Notre Dame Press.

Merleau-Ponty, Maurice (1942/1963). *The Structure of Behavior.* (A. Fisher, Trans.). Boston: Beacon Press.

———. (1945/1962). *Phenomenology of Perception* (C. Smith, Trans.). New York: Humanities Press.

———. (1964). *The Primacy of Perception* (J. Edie, Ed.). Evanston, IL: Northwestern University Press.

———. (1964/1968). *The Visible and the Invisible* (Alfonso Lingis, Trans.). Evanston, IL: Northwestern University Press.

Metz, Johnnes. (1968). *The Poverty of Spirit.* Glen Rock, NJ: Newman Press.

Moran, Gabriel. (1996). *A Grammar of Responsibility.* New York: Crossroad.

Peperzak, Adriaan. (1993). *To the Other: An Introduction to the Philosophy of Emmanuel Levinas.* West Lafayette, IN: Purdue University Press.

Piliavin, J. A., and H. W. Charng. (1990). "Altruism: A Review of Recent Theory and Research." *Annual Review of Sociology* 16: 27–65.

Smith, Hedrick. (1988). *The Power Game: How Washington Works.* New York: Random House.

Rachels, James. (1993). *The Elements of Moral Philosophy,* 2nd ed. New York: McGraw-Hill.

Ricoeur, Paul. (1950/1966). *Freedom and Nature: The Voluntary and the Involuntary* (Erazim V. Kohak, Trans.). Evanston, IL: Northwestern University Press.

Ross, L., and R. Nisbett, (1991). *The Person and the Situation: Perspectives of Social Psychology*. New York: McGraw-Hill.

Rowe, J., S. Halling. E. Davies, E. Gnaulati, D. Powers, J. Van Bronkhorst, and E. Usadi, (1986, June). "Self-Forgiveness: A Phenomenological Study of Experiencing Forgiveness." Paper presented at the Fifth International Human Science Research Conference, Berkeley, CA.

Rowe, J., S. Halling, E. Davies, M. Leifer, D. Powers, and J. Van Bronkhorst. (1989). "The Psychology of Forgiving Another: A Dialogal Research Approach." In *Existential-Phenomenological Perspectives in Psychology*, edited by R. S. Valle and S. Halling. New York: Plenum, (pp. 233–44).

Sartre, Jean-Paul. (1945/1955). *No Exit and Three Other Plays*. New York: Vintage Press.

———. (1964/1965). *Situations*. (Benita Eisler, Trans.). Greenwich, CT: Fawcett Publications.

Sloterdijk, Peter. (1983/1987). *Critique of Cynical Reason* (Michael Eldred, Trans.). Minneapolis: University of Minnesota Press.

Spiegelberg, Herbert. (1965). *The Phenomenological Movement*. The Hague: Martinus Nijhoff.

Stevenson, Robert Louis. (1950). "A Child's Garden of Verse # XXIV." *Robert Louis Stevenson: Collected Poems*. London: Rupert Hart-Davis.

Strasser, Stephen. (1982). "Emmanuel Levinas (born 1906): Phenomenological Philosophy." Translated by Herbert Spiegelberg. In Spiegelberg, Editor, *The Phenomenological Movement*, 3rd ed. The Hague: Martinus Nijhoff.

———. (1969). *The Idea of a Dialogal Phenomenology*. Pittsburgh: Duquesne University Press.

Tallon, Andrew. (1995) "Nonintentional Affectivity, Affective Intentionality, and the Ethical in Levinas's Philosophy," in *Ethics as First Philosophy: The Significance of Emmanuel Levinas for Philosophy, Literature, and Religion*. New York: Routledge.

Untener, Bishop Kenneth. (1991). "The Decree to Discuss the Poor: What Was Learned." *Origins* 21.10: 164–66.

Vitz, Paul C. (1977). *Psychology as Religion*. Grand Rapids, MI: Eerdmans Publishing.

Wyschogrod, Edith. (1990). *Saints and Postmodernism*. Chicago: University of Chicago Press.

Index